FASTING

AND

MAN'S CORRECT DIET

By

R. B. PEARSON

Construction Engineer

**Certified Member American Association
of Engineers**

□ ⊔ ⊓

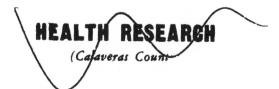

HEALTH RESEARCH
(Calaveras County)

CONTENTS

INTRODUCTION

"Is anything of God's contriving endangered by enquiry? Was it the system of the Universe or the Monks that trembled at the telescope of Galileo? Did the circulation of the firmament stop in terror because Newton laid his daring finger on its pulse?

LOWELL."

In quoting the above the present writer does not wish to imply that he is a discoverer along the lines of fasting as a perusal of the list of fasts given in Chapter 4 and a scanning of the Bibliography, incomplete as they are, will amply disprove any such idea.

However, the idea suggested by the above quotation seems appropriate in connection with the writer's attack on that old totem pole of allopathy, the germ theory. The writer's experience has satisfied him most thoroughly that germs are scavengers, that they never caused any disease whatever, and that all germs in the body, as scavengers, will die out and be eliminated just as fast as the decomposed tissue or food that they live on is consumed or removed, and he has also become convinced that the quickest and safest way to cleanse the system is by fasting and using enemas. In fact it seems almost unbelievable to the writer that, in view of the large amount of evidence that now exists that germs are scavengers, that anyone should at this late date believe otherwise.

In the writer's opinion it is utterly astonishing that the so-called "Regular" school of allopathic physicians, as represented by the American Medical Association, should be so profoundly ignorant of the laws of Nature with which they have to deal as they are at present.

The whole structure of the allopathic (A. M. A.) treatment of disease is built on absolutely false grounds.

1st. They claim germs cause disease when, in fact, it is well established that they do not, they are only Nature's scavengers of the diseased tissues and decayed food.

2nd. They claim that drugs cure disease, another claim built on absolutely false grounds as seems to have been clearly recognized by the older physicians for many years, a fact which the writer has proved to his own satisfaction by fifteen or twenty years' sad experience.

3rd. They claim that a person must continue to "eat to keep up his strength"—another fallacy as false as the first two, as has been amply proven years ago, by such authorities as Drs. Dewey, Shaw, Densmore, Haskell, Keith, Eales and Hazzard. In fact, so many allopaths' ideas on diet, in spite of their supposed "fine training" on the subject, are *absolutely false*.

It is reasonable to expect the members of a profession that pretends to be an authority on any particular subject, such as that of the treatment of disease, to receive, and consider with an open mind, the ideas of outsiders regarding their professional work, but the American Medical Association has built up a fence of license laws around their work, and refuse to consider the ideas of anyone not a graduate of a school of medicine approved by themselves. Consequently, they are almost entirely ignorant of statements of competent persons which discredit the germ theory. They are almost wholly ignorant (except a few of the older, more experienced ones) of the fact that drugs do not cure disease, and there is probably no subject whatever on which they are so completely ignorant, and so full of false ideas, as that of FASTING,—Nature's most important method of curing disease.

Perhaps all the authorities quoted above wrote with the idea of interesting the allopathic profession in fasting, as most of them were trained as allopaths themselves and took up fasting after realizing that medicine was a failure.

However, as each and every one of them has been attacked by practically the whole profession, who still hold up the germ theory as their totem pole, the present writer most sincerely hopes to reach the general public with this little book. He has not much hope of converting the allopaths but wishes to reach the general public instead, and believes the treatment of disease should be confined to such drugless schools of medicine as the Naprapaths, Osteopaths, Chiropractors, etc.: those Allopaths who believe in the germ theory, and surgery as a cure of disease, being barred from practice entirely.

If allopaths would admit they are mistaken in the 3 essential items above named, the whole structure of their learned profession would topple in the dust, hence they don't admit it, but instead try to prop it up with license laws giving them control of health departments, the exclusive treatment of disease "with or without" drugs, and allowing them through compulsory vaccination to actually commit an assault on their neighbors, with no redress for the injured party.

Hence the present author offers this volume in the hope that many "hopelessly" sick from some disease, that the allopath can't cure, such as cancer, apoplexy, paralysis, poliomye-

---

Medical Society of U. S.

Opens Convention Today

Chi. Trib. ———— 10-6-19

There will be mention of topics other than those of science when the Medical Society of the United States gathers for its fourth annual convention today at the Great Northern hotel.

The society is composed of physicians who have rebelled against the American Medical association, and that society's conduct is to be criticized.

Among speakers of the first day's session will be Dr. Ada M Chevalier of Gallup, N. M., said to have a record of saving every one of 657 influenza patients she cared for. Dr. C. A. Bryce of Richmond, Va., president, will preside, the sessions lasting three days.

litis, cerebral meningitis, tuberculosis, pneumonia, or, in fact, any and all diseases, will take up the author's ideas, without the knowledge or assistance of an allopathic physician as represented by the A. M. A. When the word allopath is used in this volume it is intended to refer only to the "germ swatters" division—the A. M. A.—as the writer does not mean such criticism to apply to such schools of medicine as may not believe in the germ theory. He was not aware of the existence of the "Medical Society of the United States," or other schools of allopaths who do not believe in the germ theory, when the book was written.

In closing the author wishes to acknowledge his own indebtedness to Dr. Hazzard and Hereward Carrington particularly, to whose books he believes he entirely owes his present fine health, and to Dr. Dewey and the other pioneers who so clearly blazed the trail for others to follow. He also begs the reader's indulgence as to any inaccuracies that may be found, the book being written largely in evenings and spare moments, in hope it might serve merely as a stepping stone to better health to many who like himself have suffered for years from ill health without getting aid from the so-called "regular" physicians.

As he is not a licensed physician and has no medical training, he would prefer not to undertake the guidance of cases of fasting himself, but would refer those who wish medical advice to Dr. L. B. Hazzard of Los Angeles or Dr. I. J. Eales of Chicago, who are both very competent authorities on the subject of fasting, or in case these parties cannot be easily reached would generally advise the reader to seek a drugless doctor when in need of advice rather than a "regular" allopath. He also wishes to acknowledge many suggestions and much help in proof-reading from Mr. John Maxwell and other friends too numerous to mention.

Chicago, July, 1921.   R. B. Pearson.

Fasting and Man's Correct Diet

CHAPTER I.

THE WRITER'S EXPERIENCE WITH CATARRH. EARLIER EFFORTS TO FIND A CURE.

There is no form of ill-health so universal, probably, as catarrh, which afflicts in some form by far the larger proportion of Americans. It is also probably in its earlier stages or milder forms, the easiest of all diseases to cure, if properly treated.

During childhood the writer had rather poor health and eyesight, also a ravenous appetite which gradually increased in intensity. At the age of thirteen a physician recommended a trip west for his health, which, however, had no effect. At this time he had a bad case of nasal catarrh and was in a run-down, neurasthenic condition, probably from catarrh of the stomach, although this was not discovered by a doctor until eight years later.

At the age of fifteen he was eating probably over 5,000 calories of food a day and still was always hungry. His right ear closed up from catarrh in the eustachian tube at this time, and a patent medicine which he tried gave such great relief from the nasal catarrh that he supposed it would cure him soon and did nothing further to open the ear. A few months after becoming deaf he had an attack of typhoid fever, which left him in a weaker condition than ever. This condition continued several years, gradually growing worse, but so slowly that he did not realize the fact, until the left ear also closed up from catarrh of the eustachian tube, about eight years later, while he was attending school in a damp climate.

He then went to a physician who said that his deafness was due to catarrh, also that the patent medicine he had been using contained morphine. However, the doctor did not say that he had any more than catarrh of the head, and paid no attention apparently to his general health, although he was in a very run-down condition, only weighing a hundred and twenty-one pounds at the age of twenty-two. The only treatment he was given was "Dobell's Solution" for use in the nose. This is merely an astringent and weak palliative, and is absolutely worthless on a severe case of catarrh which, of course, will also affect other organs than the nose. On stopping the use of the patent medicine he grew considerably weaker, and his nasal catarrh became so bad as to cause some fear of suffocating in his sleep for several weeks following.

Consequently he decided to try another physician. This doctor told him that not only was his deafness due to catarrh, but that he also had catarrh of the stomach, and that catarrh was in his blood and all through his system. This physician treated him several months, during which time his left ear was opened and his general health considerably improved. But the attempt to cure his catarrh was not successful and he was finally dismissed, the doctor having done all that he could for him.

He continued to use the medicines prescribed for some months in the hope of more improvement, and of opening the other ear, but finally decided to let an eye and ear specialist who had treated his eyes in the past, see what could be done. The two physicians of whom we have already spoken were regular allopathic physicians, the first, a man of national prominence, the second, very well recommended.

The eye and ear specialist to whom he now applied, pooh-poohed the idea that catarrh had anything to do with the deafness, claiming that hardening of the wax in the ear was the cause and opened it by digging out the hardened wax. However, it was soon deaf again and was subject to catarrhal deaf spells lasting from a few minutes to three months at a time for about nine years more, until cleared up by fasting. The left ear was also deaf at times, but the attacks were usually short.

When these deaf spells came on after the right ear had been opened, the writer concluded that physicians did not know much about catarrh, and he did not go back to the man who had opened the right ear. Instead he began reading everything he could find on the subject, with the idea of finding and removing the cause of catarrh completely.

During all the above treatment not a doctor asked a question about what he ate, or how much he ate, nor did any of them say a word that could be construed as advice to change his ways of eating, or to restrict his food in any way. Consequently he kept up the old way of eating until his appetite was fully satisfied, which took about 4,500 to 5,000 calories of food a day.

In his first attempt to cure his catarrh himself he turned to physical culture, spending a year or two on it. This not giving success in that time, he gave it up and decided to try changes in his diet. The first thing he did was to cut out meat entirely, which caused a slight improvement in health and completely cured him of boils which had troubled him for some years. But his catarrh did not seem to improve much. As a substitute for meat he used nuts, eggs and beans, also "Plasmon," a patented proteid food made from milk, but ate too much of these, hence the small improvement.

CHAPTER II.

THE WRITER'S EXPERIENCE WITH FASTING TO CURE CATARRH.

Looking further for relief he found Hereward Carrington's book, "Fasting, Vitality and Nutrition," and realized for the first time that his catarrh must be due to overeating. This was the first hint he had received that his catarrh could be due to that cause. None of the doctors consulted had given any idea of this, had they known it; nor had they given any opinion as to what they thought was the cause.

Some years before (1903-4) he had tried to fast after reading of Dr. Tanner's forty-day fast to cure rheumatism, but had given it up after sixty miserable hours, through fear of starving to death. This time he decided to try again with the book as a guide. However, the first two days brought such weakness, misery, lassitude and headaches that he gave it up again and lived on one meal a day for six months, not taking more than the equivalent of one pound of solid food a day, by weight. This caused considerable improvement in his condition, but he was still a long way from being cured. He had lost about eight pounds during the dieting, and gained about fifteen pounds in the first three days after resuming a heavier diet.

However, he soon found that the catarrhal condition was returning, and decided to take a number of short fasts of about a week or ten days each, separated by a week or two of eating 2,500 calories a day, which his reading had indicated was necessary to support life. This was kept up for several months in an irregular manner due to a weak will, which frequently lost all control over what was eaten for weeks at a time. Although he had never been hungry since the first time he fasted over three days, the odor of a savory meal after a few days fasting, seemed to arouse a desire to enjoy the taste of it. This was a sensation entirely distinct from hunger, a desire apparently of the nerves for excitement, probably very similar to a drunkard's desire for liquor. While he almost invariably over-ate between fasts due to this weakness of will power, he found that his fasting finally almost cured his catarrh. His general health was better, and his tongue, which had become very heavily coated on starting to fast, was two-thirds clear, only about one-third along the center remaining coated with the same heavy coat as it had at first. This convinced him that he had carried the fasting far enough, and had better begin to eat, as he expected the slight amount of catarrh still left would soon leave him. Consequently he started eating about 2,500 calories of food a day. The result of this was that in a few months he had catarrh again about as bad as ever.

But this had given more complete relief than anything else he had tried. Therefore he decided to make another attempt to obtain a complete cure by fasting, thinking that he had probably eaten too much after the fast, although he carefully weighed all food and knew that he was keeping close to 2,500 calories a day. He also obtained Dr. Hazzard's book, "Fasting for the Cure of Disease," about this time.

During the entire time he was following this regimen, he took enemas daily, whether fasting or eating, and found them of considerable help as the bowels generally will not move during a fast without such help; or unless a cathartic is used. There are several things to pay attention to in taking enemas. The most important of these is the temperature of the water. It should be BELOW the temperature of the blood, and not above it. Water which is warmer than the blood will, in most cases, so weaken the bowels that they will not move naturally afterwards, making a continuance of the enemas necessary indefinitely.

However, one application of an enema with the water at
80 degrees F. has repeatedly restored the bowels to full
normal vigor, even when the warmer water had been used
for some time. It is the writer's opinion that an antiseptic
should be dissolved in each enema taken, as the large quantity of water introduced into a bowel filled with putrefying
or fermenting material causes an immediate transfusion of
the toxins and other poisons to the system, where they may
cause headaches and other signs of autointoxication. Probably the best antiseptic for this purpose is baking soda. A
teaspoonful or two in a three-quart enema is about the
right amount to use. At first he used the plain water enemas about four or five times a day for eight or ten days,
gradually reducing the number of times a day it was used
as the bowels were cleaned out, until near the end of the
fast it was only being used about once a day.

Because of the help he had received from this fasting
he concluded to try again. So far he had followed the
recommendations in Carrington's and Dr. Hazzard's books
quite closely, except that he *had not kept up the fasting
until the tongue was completely cleared up,* but had stopped
fasting with still a third of the tongue covered with a heavy
coat, because he had read some place that the stomach
would fail completely if a fast was carried too far.

The second fast progressed in very much the same
manner as the first, except that conditions generally were
more favorable than during the former fast. The bowels
and, in fact, the whole system were not so foul as they had
been during the first fast. Consequently he did not feel
the weakening effects of the poisons in the system to quite
such an extent as he had the first time, and as his will was
somewhat stronger than it had been before he reached the
point where the tongue became almost clear in considerably
shorter time. Here he again stopped because he had found
that the stomach apparently could not stand a prompt re-

sumption of the ordinary diet after a fast, and he thought that by the time he could get its capacity up to normal again the catarrh or what was left of it would be gone; or that the system would be able to throw off the remaining signs of it after he began to eat what he thought was the "minimum" diet of about 2,400 calories a day. He reasoned that 2,500 calories was too high because his catarrh returned while eating that much after the first fast, hence the smaller amount. Later complete fasts taken in 1914, fall and winter, and in 1918, convinced the writer that the stomach is very much stronger if not fed until hunger returns and the tongue clears, than when fed before Nature calls for food.

However, in four or five months he found that the catarrh had again returned, apparently as bad as ever, and concluded that the trouble must be in either the quantity or kind of food eaten after the fast, as improvement had been regular and continuous as long as he fasted.

Therefore he decided to keep at it, and repeated the experiment four or five times, fasting for a week or ten days at a time and following it by a few days of eating. This was continued until the tongue was two-thirds or more cleared up, when he would resume eating until he again became weak and run-down from catarrh, which usually took several months. Each time he repeated this he reduced the amount of food eaten slightly, until he was down to about 2,000 calories a day, at the end of the seventh series of short fasts. At this time after a spell of three months, his deafness left him permanently and his health was better than it had been for over twenty years.

About two years previous to this he had found in his feces a long white ribbon about 1/8-inch thick by 5/16-inch wide and about 30 inches long, which he took for a tape worm, although he could not see any joints in it. It hung over a wire like a tape of sticky white rubber. His family physician, when he related his symptoms to him, said it might be either a tape worm or catarrh of the bowels, but on seeing a sample, declared it to be catarrh of the bowels only. This was a great relief to the author, as he felt that he could cure any kind of catarrh by fasting if he kept it up long enough. The only treatment the doctor recommended for it was the use of enemas with one or two teaspoonfuls of baking soda in three quarts of water. He used this about two years along with the fasting, and found that it reduced the catarrhal condition about 25 per cent below what it would be without the baking soda, but did not seem to have any greater effect than this. All prior fasts had been accompanied with plain water enemas only.

About the time he discovered this catarrh of the bowels he read a book on disorders of digestion, entitled "The Stomach" (published in 1896) by Dr. J. H. Kellogg, in which the author, perhaps, gives the most thorough discussion of the subject that was ever written. In this book he says among other things:

"The stomach must certainly be regarded as the center of the nutritive process of the body, and any derangement of its functions must therefore result in disorder of the entire organism.

"It may truly be said that disorders of digestion are most prevalent of all human ills, and investigators within the last twenty years (pub. 1896) have been making more and more clear the fact that the great majority of diseases are primarily due to derangement of the digestive processes. The remarkable researches of Professor Bouchard of Paris, and others, have shown that such diseases as consumption, typhoid fever, and cholera, as well as Bright's disease and analogous maladies, are indirectly, if not directly, due to a disordered condition of the stomach, as the result of which the defenses of the body are broken down, and infection rendered possible.

"The function of a tissue or an organ depends upon its structure; and the structure of every cell and fiber of the body is dependent upon the quality and quantity of the material absorbed from the alimentary canal. A deficient supply of food weakens the structure and lessens the energy of the organ. *An excess of food overwhelms the tissues with imperfectly oxidized and toxic substances, whereby their structure is deteriorated, and their functions perverted or retarded. Food containing toxic substances produces in the body general or specific toxic effects. The same thing results from the development of toxic substances in the alimentary canal from the fermentation or putrefaction of food in the stomach and intestines.*

"Many persons suffer from disorders of digestion without being aware of the fact. Headache, backache, bladder and kidney disorders, sleeplessness, depression of spirits, weakness, lack of energy, coldness of the extremities, nervous sensations of various sorts, even hysteria, epilepsy, and insanity, may exist as the result of indigestion without any suffering in the stomach, or anything to suggest to the patient himself or to the untrained observer, any disorder of digestion. In every case of chronic disease, the stomach should be carefully investigated. A coated tongue is always indicative of a disordered stomach. The same is true of numerous other symptoms from which many people suffer, such as a bad taste in the mouth, dullness or headache after eating, nervous headache, etc.

Pg. 80. "*Overeating*—Intemperance in eating is in the opinion of the writer, responsible for a greater amount of evil in the world than is intemperance in drink, and also that it is one of the obstacles in the way of the reformation of those who have become the victims of alcoholic intemperance.

Pg. 82. "Excessive eating also occasions injury to the health by producing an excessive fullness of the blood-vessels, thus incurring the risk of rupture within the brain, and resulting paralysis. Other equally serious mischiefs may arise from the accumulation in the system of a greater quantity of nutritive material than can be utilized, which occasions general clogging and obstruction of all the bodily functions, and imposes an enormous burden upon the kidneys in the elimination of the unusable material.

After the later fasts when he again began eating, he felt very comfortable for a few days, then had a full feeling as though the blood pressure was increasing; this would be followed in a day or two by a severe nose bleed impossible to stop until the pressure was reduced; after which he would very soon grow dull and stupid with a return of his catarrh gradually increasing in its intensity until it was as bad as ever. Owing to the rapidity with which these events followed each other, it took several repetitions to convince him that he was grossly overeating, even at 2,000 calories a day.

In looking about for further information as to the minimum diet, he found in Upton Sinclair's book on fasting, that a young lady friend of Mr. Sinclair had lived on 1,200 calories a day, although Mr. Sinclair himself appeared to have gone through the same experience as the writer, of alternating fasting with such heavy overeating that he soon had to fast again to clean out his system.

About the end of the seventh series of fasts, in February, 1914, the writer left an office position and took an outside job on construction work, thinking that he had completely cured his catarrh; and because of the heavier work went back to eating 2,500 calories a day. After six months of this work and diet he found he was losing weight fast. The catarrh had returned in full force, in fact, was worse apparently than it had been since the first fast; but it did not have nearly as much effect in the head. There was no deafness and the nasal catarrh was extremely light.

However what was lacking in catarrh in the head was fully made up by more severe catarrhal conditions in the body than he had experienced before. The stomach reached a point before he realized it, where it could not digest sufficient nourishment to replace the daily wear and tear of the body. The urinary tract became stopped up with catarrhal mucus to such an extent that it was almost impossible to urinate until the bladder was full, and he was in the most run-down sickly condition he had been in since the first fast.

He became satisfied it would be necessary to fast until his tongue cleared up, regardless of a warning he had read somewhere that during too long a fast, the stomach would fail completely, and he also decided to hold the amount of nourishment taken after the fast, down to the least that would support life, if he could find any means of telling what that was. Both H. Carrington and Dr. Linda B. Hazzard say in their books on fasting that *natural hunger will come to persons who fast until their systems are clean,* and he had not yet experienced any such feeling after prior fasts because he had not fasted until the tongue was clear. He had read in medical works that the tongue will have about the same thickness of coating as prevails throughout the mucus membrane lining the interior organs of the body, and hence indicates their condition quite clearly.

This fast came during the business slump in the winter of 1914-15, hence he was able to drop everything and give it his whole attention. For the first few months it progressed very much as the former series of fasts, generally about ten days of fasting, alternating with a week, or two or three, of more or less hearty eating which varied widely with the conditions of the will and the urging of friends to eat. However, he finally came to the point where he had broken off prior fasts. He was quite thin. His tongue was two-thirds clear with the middle third heavily coated. At this point he ate for a few days and then proceeded to finish the fast with another ten-day stretch, at the end of which he found his stomach had gone out of business entirely, as far as digestion was concerned.

He tried everything he could think of, not exceeding an ounce of food a day, but it all lay on the stomach like a lump of lead; butter, peanut butter, raw egg, milk, etc.; items which had been the most easily digested substances in the past; all remained in the stomach for days without apparent change. This continued for twenty-five or thirty days. At the end of this time he felt a slight twitching at the back of one knee joint where he had had a soft tumerous growth for about twenty years, and found this growth completely gone. The tongue also cleared up, his eyesight became very clear, and peristaltic action suddenly set in, in the stomach. The lump in the stomach was carried off and he found that he could eat, and seemed able to digest considerable food, and do it rapidly.

During the last twenty-five or thirty days he had been extremely weak. At times it took several efforts to get up out of a chair. His legs would go to sleep while sitting comfortably, and his knees were wobbly when he walked. He was also very short of breath when he did anything, although he breathed more rapidly and deeply than usual, all day long. During nearly the entire fast, large quantities of catarrhal mucus came out with the foulest excrement. The mucus looked exactly like small sheets of transparent skin about an inch square, but had no more cohesiveness when picked up on a wire, than so much slime. This he took to be ample proof that it was mucus and not membrane. This stopped coming out just before the peristaltic action started up, and the excreta became perfectly odorless.

At the end of this fast the writer found himself absolutely free from catarrh for probably the first time in his life, and with the cleanest system he had ever had. During the later intervals between the fasts he found that an enema and a little fasting would entirely cure the toothache, due to lack of attention to cavities in the teeth, and towards the end of the complete fast the mouth, which had been very foul for some time, had some remarkable changes. Teeth with black cavities became white and clear, all decay seemed to be arrested by the fast, and there were no more toothaches, until the had overeaten for a considerable length of time. Furthermore, the foul taste was displaced by a very sweet, clean, pleasant taste at the end of the fast.

Another strange thing that occurred was that during the first week or two after this fast it was absolutely impossible to catch cold. No exposure that would previously have brought on a cold or sickness, had any such effect whatever. Mosquito bites which had always caused large swellings and severe itching in the past entirely lost their power to do so. They did not cause any swelling, inflammation or itch whatever, until he had again begun to overeat. Even hornet stings which in the past had caused severe inflammation lasting a considerable length of time, did not cause any inflammation, swelling or itch. Wouldn't this clearing up of the decaying teeth and the lack of results from mosquito and hornet bites and exposure to colds indicate that germs were losing their hold?

The first week after the fast was broken the writer lived on about two ounces of sweet chocolate and two ounces of peanuts, and one or sometimes two chocolate malted milks at a soda fountain, per day. This constituted about four ounces of solid food or about 1,000 calories a day, which is much below the "Voigt" standard of 2,500 calories a day. On this diet the bowels moved regularly about two hours after eating and seemed very energetic, and the excrement had no odor whatever.

However, after a week or ten days of this low diet he feared it was insufficient to support life and decided to increase it from four to six ounces of solid food a day, the result being that the excrement immediately took on the odor of the food eaten, while in about a week fermentation set in in the bowels, and gradually increased in degree until another series of fasts was taken. This was believed to indicate that six ounces of food a day was more than was required to nourish a man of approximately 150 pounds, while doing office work.

The fact that the excrement had no odor during the first week after the longer fast, was taken as an indication that this might be the proper condition for the bowels at all times; although the amount eaten seemed extremely small to sustain life permanently. The writer had read H. Fletcher's book, "The A B-Z of Our Nutrition," years before, but had utterly failed to attain odorless excrement at that time.

The following four years were spent experimenting on diet trying to find a diet that would give all the nourishment and strength needed and still be free from the toxins that would cause a return of the catarrh. Several times the author thought he had found a good diet, only to find in a few months of it that the catarrhal conditions were coming back, indicating overeating.

Finally in 1918 when his catarrh had again become rather severe through overeating, especially in the stomach, bowels and urinary system, he again took a series of short fasts to clean out his system and again reached a condition where his natural hunger returned, tongue cleared up, excreta became odorless, and the catarrh completely disappeared. Apparently all germ activity also disappeared with the catarrh.

The writer has gone into considerable detail as to his experience, having felt it necessary to show substantial grounds for the conclusions he has come to, and the absolute necessity of sanitary measures in treating disease; and also in hope that it may serve to assist others in the same condition to avoid many of the blunders he at first made, although he does not wish to imply that he has been through any real suffering. Catarrh is a comparatively harmless trouble, and though hard to cure, it seldom kills.

The discussion of the conclusions drawn from the fasts and the writer's idea of the correct diet for an adult will be taken up in later chapters.

CHAPTER III.

CONCLUSIONS FROM THE RESULT OF FASTING FOR CATARRH, AND A DISCUSSION OF THE CAUSE OF DISEASE.

The strange effect the final fast had of apparently destroying germ action, and rendering the system immune to germ attack, together with the fact that the supposed effects of germs had varied so much during the long series of fasts, always decreasing during the fast and increasing while eating, except during the short time the writer ate so little that the excreta had no odor, led the writer to believe that germs must be the result of disease, or scavengers of diseased tissue as suggested by Dr. Dewey rather than the cause; and that the cause of disease must be almost entirely a overeating. While all physiologists argue that germs are the cause of disease rather than merely scavengers, in the writer's opinion their ideas are founded on false grounds.

For instance, it is clearly recognized that nearly all bacteria found in nature outside the body are scavengers only, as note the statement in "Americana" under "Bacteria."

Contrary to notions that have been more or less prevalent the majority of bacteria have nothing to do with disease production. Their natural role is that of scavengers. They are concerned in nature's great laboratory, the soil, in working over dead organic matters into forms appropriate to the nourishment of growing vegetation. Since in the course of this conversion dead bodies that would otherwise encumber the earth are caused to disappear they must from both the aesthetic and economic standpoints be regarded as, in the main, benefactors. In this group of *saprophytic* bacteria, as they are called, that is, *those that live on dead matters*, we encounter species of the greatest interest and importance. It is here that we perceive the omnipresent forms concerned in the reduction of dead animal and vegetable tissues into such simple forms as carbon dioxide, ammonia and water to be

used by higher plants. It is in this group that we find the
ever present nitrifying species—that is, those peculiar ferments
that . . . . . . convert the objectionable organic
matters of sewage and polluted waters into an inert inorganic
form. . . . . . . The evil odors of putrefaction are
the results of saprophytic bacterial development.

This may be true, but the writer holds that the putrefaction itself is not the result of bacterial action, but is
purely chemical, a form of decay for which these bacteria
are the natural scavengers. Furthermore we find practically full recognition of the fact it is a chemical process,
although this is in turn ascribed to bacterial action in
"Elem. Biology" by T. J. Parker (p. 90), where he say.. in
discussing the nutrition of bacteria:

". . . nearly all of those to which reference has been
made are saprophytes, that is, live upon decomposing animal
and vegetable matters,"
and then he goes on to ascribe fermentation to bacterial
action and on the next page he says:

"Putrefaction itself is another instance of fermentation
induced by a microbe. Bacterium termo—the putrefactive ferment—causes the decomposition of proteids into simpler com-
pounds, amongst which are such gases as ammonia (NH_3),
sulphuretted hydrogen (H_2S) and ammonium sulphide
($(NH_4)_2S$), the evolution of which produces the characteristic
odor of putrefaction.

The final stage in putrefaction is the formation of nitrates
and nitrites. The process is a double one, both stages being
due to special forms of bacteria. In the first place, by the
agency of the nitrous ferment, ammonia is converted into
nitrous acid:

$$NH_3 + 3O = H_2O + HNO_2$$
Ammonia Oxygen Water Nitrous acid

The nitric ferment then comes into action, converting the
nitrous into nitric acid:

$$NHO_2 + O = NHO_3$$
Nitrous acid Oxygen Nitric acid

This process is of vast importance, since by its agency
the soil is constantly receiving fresh supplies of nitric acid,

which is one of the most important substances used as food by plants."

Now, why can't these be considered common, ordinary chemical reactions induced by the slow or moderate heat of summer. Also what would happen if these bacteria should be unavailable when wanted? Would not a chemist have to send out to borrow a few?.

On page 93 he goes on to say:

"As to temperature, common observation tells us that bacteria flourish only within certain limits. We know for instance that organic substances can be preserved from putrefaction by being kept either at the freezing point or at or near the boiling point. . . . Similarly it is a matter of common observation that a moderately high temperature is advantageous to these organisms, the heat of summer or the tropics being notoriously favorable to putrefaction. . . ."

In Thorpe's "Dictionary of Applied Chemistry," Vol. 2, p. 502, under "Fermentation," after discussing and accepting the bacterial causation theory for same it notes:

". . . Many difficulties, however, still remained unexplained, which prevented the universal acceptance of the vitalistic view (bacterial cause). Milk, for example, was found to become sour after having been boiled, in spite of all precautions, and no organism could be recognized in it capable of producing the change."

Now, if bacteria were not present at this time, hence could not have caused the milk to sour for this time at least, why not believe that their presence at other times might only be accidental, or in the capacity of scavengers for the decomposing material?

The first authority, "Americana" Ency., under the heading of Bacteriology, says:

"As a result of these studies (modern bacteriology) we know that sewage, polluted waters and polluted soils tend naturally to revert to a state of purity if their pollution be checked and that this progressive purification is due in large part to the activities of the bacteria located within them."

But in the first article Bacteria, he goes on to say, discussing the bacteria found within the body:

"In the parasitic group of bacteria we encounter those species that exist always at the expense of a living host, either animal or vegetable, and in doing so not only appropriate materials necessary to life, but give off in return waste products that may act as direct poisons to the host. Fortunately, this is a much smaller group than is the saprophytic mentioned above. *In no particulars, save for their ability to exist at the expense of a living host and cause disease are the disease-producing bacteria distinguishable from the innocent varieties. The essential difference between the disease-producing and the innocent bacteria species is that the former possess as their most striking physiological peculiarity the power of elaborating poisons, toxins, technically speaking, that have a direct destructive action upon the tissues of their host.*"

Isn't this strange? Only one kind of bacteria are accused of forming poisons while all others are said to destroy poisons wherever found.

Now how do they know that bacteria cause or produce these toxins or have any hand in doing this? The Ency. Brit., Vol. 3, p. 172, says under "Bacteriology-Cultivation":

"In cultivating bacteria outside the body various media to serve as food material must be prepared and sterilized by heat. The general principle in their preparation is to supply the nutriment for bacterial growth in a form as nearly similar as possible to that of the natural habitat, the natural fluids of the body. . . . . To mention examples *blood-serum solidified at a suitable temperature is a highly suitable medium, and various media are made with extract of meat as a basis, with the addition of gelatine or agar as solidifying agents and of non-coagulable proteids (commercial "peptone") to make up for proteids lost by coagulation in the preparation.* . . . . . For most purposes the solid media are to be preferred, since bacterial growth appears in a discrete mass and accidental contamination can be readily recognized. Cultures are made by transferring by means of a sterile platinum wire a little of the material containing the bacteria to the medium. The tubes, after being thus inoculated, are kept at suitable temperatures, usually either 37 C., the temperature of the body, or at about 20 C., a warm summer temperature. *until growth appears.*"

Now Bouchard says that when meat is held in the digestive tract in the body over 5 hours the changes that take place are putrefactive rather than digestive, or in other words, decomposition begins after 5 hours at this heat in the body. Does it appear reasonable to suppose that any meat tissues, any blood-serum, or any "extract of meat" could remain at this heat outside the body any greater length of time without decomposition setting in, especially when we remember that the digestive juices are all considered destructive to both germs and toxins? No, of course not. The meat or proteids in these blood serums or "extracts of meat" are rapidly decomposed by the heat, hence hen the bacteria are planted thereon they find it "easy picking" and multiply like flies in a manure pile.

It seems very strange to the writer that toxins found in such a solution after the bacteria begin to grow should be considered the work of the bacteria; why not try keeping a few "preparations" at this temperature *without inoculation with bacteria,* and see if they don't decompose just as fast and produce just as much "toxin" material as the preparations inoculated with bacteria?

The Ency. Brit., Vol. 3, p. 172d, under Bacteriology, says:

"As our knowledge has advanced it has become abundantly evident that the so-called pathogenic bacteria are not organisms with special features, but that each is a member of a group of organisms possessing closely allied characters. From the point of view of evolution we may suppose that certain races of a group of bacteria have gradually acquired the power of invading the tissues of the body and producing disease. In the acquisition of pathogenic properties some of their original characters have become changed, *but in many instances this has taken place only to a light degree, and furthermore, some of these changes are not of a permanent char-*

acter. It is to be noted that in the case of bacteria we can
only judge of organisms being of different species by the stability of the characters which distinguish them and *numerous
examples might be given where their characters become modified by comparatively slight change in their environment. The
cultural as well as the microscopical characters of a pathogenic
organism may be closely similar to other non-pathogenic members of the same group, and it thus becomes a matter of extreme difficulty in certain cases . . . . . in differentiating varieties."*

Don't this look as if someone was getting a little fud-
dled up in their reasoning?

First, they say the pathogenic (toxin producing) bacteria are so much like the non-pathogenic (non-toxin producing) kind that they can only be told apart by the power
to produce toxins, in fact, they actually believe that certain
"races" of bacteria acquire toxin-producing powers and
then turn around and lose them, a sort of diminutive
"magician" as it were. Isn't it far easier to believe the
toxins are merely decayed tissue or food, and the bacteria
merely scavengers living on these toxins wherever they find
any?

In Good Health and How We Won It, by Upton
Sinclair and Michael Williams, the statement is made that
one of the authors in taking treatment and change of diet
at the Battle Creek Sanitarium reduced the number of
microbes (the "dangerous" bacterial inhabitants of the intestinal tract) from 4 billion per gram of intestinal con-
tents nearly 90 per cent.

Now why did these 90 per cent leave or die just because of a six weeks' change from a meat (toxic) to a non-
toxic diet, especially if they could "have a direct destructive
action upon the tissues of their host?" The writer believes
these germs were living on the toxins formed from the putrefaction of the meat in the system and died off when this
(the real) source of the toxins was lost. His own experi-

ence in the excrement becoming odorless at the end of long
fasts bears this view out completely.

The New Int. Ency., Vol. 7, p. 68, says under "Diseases, Germ Theory of":

"Then, too, the body is so built as to offer very powerful
resistance to the entrance into it of most germs. First in
importance of the body defenses against germ invasion is the
skin. The unbroken skin offers an almost impassable barrier
to the passage of most forms of germs.

"Being the most exposed it is also the strongest of the
body defenses against the entrance into it of micro-organisms.
Few if any germs have the power to penetrate it if healthy
and intact."

Describing the internal organs it says:

"These openings and tracts are lined by mucous membranes which may be considered as forming a second line
f defence against germ invasion. Being less exposed than
.he skin, the mucous membranes are also less resistant than
the skin to the entrance of germs. Indeed, to certain species
of germs the mucous membranes are especially susceptible;
as the mucous membrane of the intestine to the bacillus of
typhoid fever, that of the respiratory tract to the diphtheria
bacillus and to the bacillus of pneumonia, and that of the
genito-urinary tract to the gonococcus."

Notice this, it is only in the *organs of elimination*
where the decomposing food materials would be carried by
the blood in the natural course of life that germs have any
chance at all to "make a living." This is just what would
be expected if it were acknowledged that germs were scavengers.

The writer's experience during his fasts has convinced
him that it is only when putrefaction and fermentation and
their products are present in the bowels and other organs
that germs can exist there at all; in other words, when his
excrement is perfectly odorless, as occurs at the end of a
properly conducted fast, he appears in every way immune
to germ action of various kinds, as is clearly shown by the
fact that at this time the bites of insects such as mosquitoes

or hornets *never* cause any swelling, any itch or any inflammation: all of which *always* occurs from this cause when putrefaction is present in the bowels. It also seems impossible to catch colds or any illness of any kind when free from putrefaction and fermentation in the digestive tract.

Now let's look further among the Encyclopædias on the subject:

In Nelson's Ency., Vol. 6, p. 5190, under Bacteria, it says:

"In practically all the bacterial diseases of man the infective agent is discharged in one or other of the excretions of the body; and the germs being adapted especially to the fluids of the body, die out more or less rapidly in the world outside."

It is far more likely to say that they die out when the toxins that they live on and that were excreted with then are consumed.

In Enc. Brit., Vol. 3, p. 173, it says:

". . . . . it may now be stated as an accepted fact that all the important results of bacteria in the tissues are due to the poisonous bodies or toxins formed by them."

Further on it says after discussing various experiments such as injecting toxic fluids from which all bacteria have been filtered into animals, that (p. 173)

"In other words, the toxins of different bacteria are closely similar in their results on the body and the features of the corresponding diseases are largely regulated by the vital properties of the bacteria, their distribution in the tissues, etc."

On the next page, 174a, he says:

"*Not only are the general symptoms of poisoning in bacterial disease due to toxic substances, but also the tissue changes, many of them of inflammatory nature, in the neighborhood of bacteria.*"

On page 173d he says in discussing experiments in which certain bacteria failed to produce toxins or anything giving toxic action outside the body:

"This and similar facts have suggested that some toxins are only produced in the living body."

In the Ency. Brit., Vol. 3, p. 174d, he says:

"A bacterial infection when analyzed is seen to be of the nature of an intoxication. There is, however, another all-important factor concerned, viz., the multiplication of the living organisms in the tissues; this is essential to, and regulates, the supply of toxins."

Would not the bacteria multiply faster on a larger supply of toxins than on a small supply if they were scavengers?

You wouldn't say that the faster flies multiplied around a garbage pile the larger it grew, would you? It is no more reasonable to say that the faster the bacteria multiply, the more toxins we have in the body. It is a result, not the cause, of the larger supply of toxins.

Aren't there a good many discrepancies in this series of arguments?

1st. There is said to be no distinguishable difference between the disease-producing bacteria in the body and the scavenger bacteria found in the ground, except the ability to produce toxins or poisons that "destroy the host."

Next, neither the bacteria or toxins can destroy the skin, unless injured, nor do they seem to have much effect on the mucous membrane except in the organs of elimination where any poisons or toxins in the body would naturally be carried by the blood. Next, they die off at the rate of 90 per cent in 6 weeks if you quit eating meat, and also die more or less rapidly if eliminated from the body in the excrement. Next we find it is not the bacteria that cause disease, but the toxins and the bacteria merely regulate the "features" of the disease.

Lastly, but not least, "some" of these bacteria which produce these toxins within the body seem to be unable to produce the same toxins outside the body. Why is this? and what are these terrible toxins, anyway?

The Ency. Brit., Vol. 3, p. 174, says:

"Regarding the chemical nature of toxins less is known than regarding the physiological action. Though an enormous amount of work has been done on the subject, no important bacterial toxin has as yet been obtained in a pure condition, and though many of them are probably of a proteid nature, even this cannot be asserted with absolute certainty. . . . . . The general result of such research has been to show that the toxic bodies are like proteids, precipitable by alcohol and various salts; they are soluble in water, and somewhat easily dialysable, and are relatively unstable both to light and heat. Attempts to get a pure toxin by repeated precipitation and solution have resulted in the production of a whitish amorphous powder with highly toxic properties. *Such a powder gives a proteid reaction, and is no doubt largely composed of albumoses*, hence the name 'tox-albumosis' has been applied."

Proteid—where did we hear that word before—isn't meat proteid? Could not these toxins come from meat? Chittenden says we all eat too much proteid food. Bouchard says that when food remains in the stomach more than 5 hours the action that takes place ceases to be of a digestive nature and becomes putrefactive and fermentative. If these toxins are merely decayed meat, of course the organs of elimination would be where they would most likely be found. Also, these same organs seem to be the only place bacteria can get into the system. Also, the bacteria seem to die very rapidly when the "host" quits a meat diet for a Battle Creek or "non-toxic" diet. Why? If these bacteria can produce toxins that "destroy the host, why don't they go ahead and destroy him just the same on a non-toxic diet? Why do 90 per cent of such "strong" germs die in 6 weeks? Don't these facts point very clearly to the idea that the toxins come from decayed food and the bacteria have the same role of scavenger in the body as they have outside?

Where do they get the idea that bacteria produce these

toxins or that bacteria cause disease, and how do they account for the above facts?

In Ency. Brit., Vol. 3, p. 158, under Bacteriology, it says:

"Long before any clear ideas as to the relations of Schizomycetes to fermentation and disease were possible various thinkers at different times had suggested that resemblances existed between the phenomena of certain diseases and those of fermentation, and the idea that a virus or contagium might be something of the nature of a minute organism capable of spreading and reproducing itself had been entertained."

Why bring in the minute organism? You note that one so-called scientist will tell you fermentation and disease are caused by bacteria, while another says, "Sewage tends to clarify itself by bacterial action." Fermentation is not caused by any minute organism, but is purely chemical in nature, a decay of animal or vegetable tissue, the products of which are consumed by bacteria within the body as well as in the soil and the fact that the "phenomena of certain diseases" resembled those of fermentation is no indication that these diseases were due to any bacteria, but, in fact, really indicates that these "certain diseases" may be the result of the fermentation or may even be the same thing as the fermentation developed under slightly different conditions than fermentation outside the body.

The article quoted continues:

"Such vague notions began to take more definite shape as the ferment theory of Cazniard de la Tour (1828), Schwan (1857) and Pasteur made way, especially in the hands of the last named savant.

"From about 1870 onwards the germ theory has passed into acceptance. P. F. O. Rayer in 1850 and Davaine had observed the bacilli in the blood of animals dead of anthrax (splenic fever), and Pollender discovered them anew in 1855. In 1863, imbued with ideas derived from Pasteur's researches on fermentation, Devaine reinvestigated the matter, and put forth the opinion that the anthrax bacilli caused the splenic fever; this was proved to result from inoculation. Koch in 1876 published his observation on Devaine's bacilli, their causal relation to splenic fever, discovered the spores and the saprophytic phase in the life history of the organism, and cleared up important points in the whole question. In 1870 Pasteur had proved that a disease of silk worms was due to an organism of the nature of a bacterium; and in 1871 Oertel showed that a micrococcus already known to exist in diphtheria is intimately concerned in producing that disease.

"Thus arose the foundations of the modern 'germ theory of disease'; and, *in the midst of the wildest conjectures and the worst of logic, a nucleus of facts was won,* which has since grown and is growing daily."

It looks to the present writer as if we still had most of the "wildest conjectures" and "worst of logic" present in modern bacteriology. If bacteria cause disease, how do you account for immunity of various degrees? Do the bacteria have sick or weak periods, or have a harmless or "tadpole" stage to go through at times?

In the New Int. Ency., Vol 12, p. 26, under "Theories of Immunity," it says:

"The exact causes of the phenomena of immunity are not well understood, but various theories have been proposed which make them more or less intelligible. In 1880 Pasteur taught that the micro-organism, by its growth in the body, uses up some substances necessary for its existence and then perishes. If the removal of this substance be complete perfect immunity results. This is the *exhaustion theory.*"

Wouldn't this account for every condition and fact before mentioned that can not be explained otherwise? The bacteria don't cause disease, it is the toxins. The bacteria merely regulate the "features" of the disease. Ninety per cent of the bacteria die off when you change from a meat to a non-toxic diet. When the writer fasts until his excrement is odorless (free from toxins), he seems to become completely immune to germ action. "Some" bacteria cannot produce toxins outside the body, etc. It accounts for all the conditions noted and all degrees of immunity in a perfectly logical manner entirely worthy of the name Pasteur.

However, it has critics, for instance, the same article, "Theories of Immunity," goes on to say:

"Sternberg combats it, saying that if it were true we must have in each of our bodies certain smallpox material, measles material, and scarlet fever material, etc., each of which must be exhausted by its appropriate micro-organism, thus necessitating an almost inconceivably complex body chemistry."

Why? Can't different kinds of bacteria live on the same kind of toxins the same as different kinds of dogs can live on one kind of meat? If this were true, wouldn't it be as necessary, very likely, for a white man to restrict himself to white meat and a colored man to live on dark meat? The present writer considers this objection totally unworthy of attention. His own experience with toxins and germs supports Pasteur's exhaustion theory in every way. The statement (p. 28) that bacteria merely regulate the features of the disease while the action of the toxins of different bacteria is much alike, also indicate this.

However, the same article gives two more theories as follows:

"The *retention theory* was advanced in 1880 by Chazveaus, who suggested that the growth of the bacteria in the body probably originated some substances prejudicial to their further development."

This might have been reasonable in 1880, but would hardly account for the remarkable decrease of germs present when anyone leaves the meat diet, nor would it account for the immunity that follows fasting to natural hunger. The same article continues:

"The *phagocytosis theory* was suggested by Carl Roser in 1881, received attention from Sternberg and also from Koch, but was not advanced with any insistence until, in 1884, Metchnikov enthusiastically championed it and gave it his name. There are two varieties of the white blood corpuscles whose duty it is to destroy bacteria:—these are the large uni-cellular leucocytes or macrophagocyte, and the smaller forms, the polymiclear leucocyte or microphagocyte. Both these forms exhibit amoeboid movements and possess the attractive force called chemotaxis which exists between amoeboid cells and food particles. Phagocytosis is the incorporation of foreign particles by those amoeboid white blood corpuscles."

The present writer will admit that white blood cor-puscles may destroy bacteria to some extent, but it is very clear that this will not account for the conditions hereto-fore noted as well as the exhaustion theory, nor will it ac-count for periodic returns of illness nor epidemics as will the exhaustion theory, nor for a person catching one dis-ease, as influenza, just after being vaccinated for another one, such as typhoid fever.

It is very plain that the theory that the bacteria ex-haust some substance on which they live (the toxins) as suggested by Pasteur, is the real explanation of their dying out in the body after an illness, and immunity for a time after a disease. It will also very clearly account for every condition noted and is in complete accord with the idea that the bacteria are scavengers in the body as well as elsewhere.

In an article entitled "Germophobia" by Helen S. Grey, in Forum for Oct. '14, she says: (p. 585)

"All the leading works of bacteriology admit that a per-son may have germs of diphtheria, typhoid fever, tuberculosis, pneumonia or any other disease within his body without hav-ing any of those diseases. Since that is the case it is obvious that germs of themselves cannot cause disease. They do no harm in a body that is in a healthy condition. But so preju-dicial is the medical profession on the subject of germs that the true causes of disease are overlooked and disregarded.

"Even some of the regulars do not hold orthodox views. for instance, Dr. Charles Creighton, an eminent English phy-sician. He has made a special study of epidemics and was engaged to write an article for the Ency. Britannica on Vaccination.

At that time he was a believer in it, but changed his views when he investigated the subject. What he wrote was omitted from the American editions. 'As a medical man,' he once declared, '*I assert that vaccination is an insult to common sense; that it is superstitious in its origin, unsatisfactory in theory and practice, and useless and dangerous in its character.*' He testified before the British Royal Commission on Vaccination that in his opinion vaccination affords no protection whatever. He has written several books on the subject.

If germs are not the cause of disease then what is? To this Dr. J. H. Tilden of Denver, one of the most distinguished of those who do not accept the germ theory of disease as true, makes answer as follows. I quote excerpts taken here and there from his writings in A Stuffed Club Magazine (now Philosophy of Health) on the subject of the causes and cure of disease, the germ theory, contagion and infection and immunity:

'Disease is brought about by obstructions and inhibitions of vital processes. . . . The basis is chronic auto-intoxication from food poisoning. It is brought about by abusing the body in many ways . . . and by living wrongly in whatever way. . . . Bad habits of living enervate . . . weaken the body and in consequence elimination is impaired. . . . The inability of the organism to rid itself of waste products brings on auto-toxemia. This systematic derangement is ready at all times to join with exciting causes to create anything from a pimple to a brain abscess and from a cold to consumption. Without this derangement, injuries and such contingent influences as are named exciting causes would fail to create disease. This is the constitutional derangement that is necessary before we can have such local manifestations as tonsilitis, pneumonia and appendicitis. . . . Every disease is looked upon as an individuality which is no more the truth than that words are made up of letters independent of the alphabet. As truly as that every word must go back to the alphabet for its letter elements *so must every disease go back to auto-toxemia for its initial elements.* . . . There can be no independent organic action in health or disease.' "

Miss Grey goes on to say:

"If drugs, serums, etc., do not cure disease, what does? Correcting whatever habits caused it, for instance, *eating too much*, bolting food, neglect of bathing, ventilation, and exercise, harboring worry, jealousy, or other destructive emotions, and living on a haphazard dietary of carelessly and ignorantly cooked foods. '*Nature cures when there is any curing done*, but nature must have help by way of removal of obstructions to normal functioning.' There is nothing spectacular about a real cure, it means self discipline. . . . *Bacteria are not the cause of disease; wrong living, which puts the system into such a condition that the bacteria can readily multiply, is the real cause;* the bacteria are simply necessary results. . . . Germs are scavengers. When an environment becomes crowded with them it means that there is a great accumulation of waste in a state of decay; . . . they are normal to a certain limit in our bodies.

If they become more numerous, common sense and reason would say that they must be a necessary factor in the process of elimination, or, if not a necessary factor, lost resistance has permitted them to multiply beyond the restrictions set to them by an ideal physical condition or normal resistance."

Additional evidence that germs do not cause disease and that sanitation has more to do with one's condition of health and immunity to disease is given by the numerous experiments made recently by army officers and others.

In Public Health Report (issued by the U. S. Public Health Service) for January 10, 1919, Vol. 34, No. 2, p. 33, is discussed some experimental efforts by medical officers of the Medical Corps, U. S. N. R. F. and the U. S. Public Health Service, at the U. S. Quarantine Station, Gallops Island, Boston, Mass., to transmit influenza from the sick to well men.

A number of different experiments were made on 68 volunteers from U. S. Naval Detention Training Camp on Deer Island.

Several groups of men (volunteers) were inoculated with pure cultures of Pfeiffer's bacillus, with secretions from the upper respiratory passages, and with blood from typical cases of influenza. About 30 men had the germs sprayed or swabbed in nose and throat. . . .

They say of the results:

"In no instance was an attack of influenza produced in any one of the subjects."

Ten more men were taken to the bedside of 10 new cases of influenza, spent 45 minutes with them, and each well man had 10 sick men cough in his face.

They say of these cases:

"None of these volunteers developed any symptoms of influenza following this experiment."

In another article the results of similar experiments in San Francisco are described.

In these experiments one group of 10 men had emulsifying cultures of Pfeiffer's bacillus with no results in 7 day's observations.

Other groups of men (40 in all) received emulsions of secretions from the upper respiratory passages of active cases of influenza which were instilled into nose by a medicine dropper or atomizer.

Of these it says:

"In every case the results were negative, so far as the reproduction of influenza is concerned. The men were all observed for seven days after inoculation."

Last, but not least, Dr. John B. Fraser, M. D. C. M., in an article entitled "Do Germs Cause Disease?" in the Physical Culture Magazine for May, 1919, says that experiments carried out in Toronto in 1911-12 and '13 proved that germs only appear *"after"* the onset of the disease, and goes on to say—

"and this fact led to the supposition that germs were simply a by-product of disease and possibly harmless."

He also describes experiments where millions of germs were fed to patients in their food, were swabbed over the tonsils and soft palate, under the tongue and in the nostrils, and still no evidence of disease was discernible.

The germs used in the experiments included the germs of diphtheria, pneumonia, typhoid fever, meningitis and tuberculosis, and no evidence of the diseases have developed in nearly 5 years.

He says:

"During the years 1914-15-16-17-18 over 150 experiments were carried out carefully and scientifically and yet absolutely no signs of disease followed."

Dr. E. H. Dewey says in "The True Science of Living" (p. 132) : (This was published in 1894.)

"In matters of external decomposition there are the crows, the buzzards, and the lesser and lesser scavengers, down to the microbes, all to enjoy the same feast. Has nature not provided for internal decomposition? There are the microbes, the non-infecting, that are the natural inhabitants of the mouth. Do not these increase because of a need? Is it not possible that the real essential cause is too subtle for the microscope, and that after all the infecting twin brothers of the native inhabitants may also act in the same sanitary sense?"

If these germs are merely scavengers, as the writer contends, then they should disappear when the toxins are eliminated, as they appear to after an illness is cured and also in the writer's and some other fasting cases. This would also account for the failure of some experimenters mentioned by Horace Fletcher in efforts to raise cultures of germs on the excreta of animals which had been held on a restricted diet of pasteurized milk and air filtered germ free, for a week. It would also account for the failures of vaccination in so large a percentage of cases.

That sanitation has an important part (if not the exclusive role) in preventing disease is indicated by the results of the reduction in the death rate after Sanitary Surveys were made by the Public Health Service in different parts of the country, principally rural districts.

For instance, a Sanitary Survey was made in Wilson county, Kansas, from April 3 to October 21, 1915, by agents of the Public Health Service who made many recommendations as to improving the sanitary conditions of isolated families.

The record of typhoid fever was:

In 1914—52 cases—7 deaths.
In 1915—26 cases—2 deaths.
In 1916—18 cases—0 deaths.

which is all ascribed to sanitation.

Again, in Public Health Report, Vol. 34, No. 13 for March 28, 1919, under the heading:

"Typhoid Vaccination no Substitute for Sanitary Precautions," a circular of the chief surgeon, A. E. F., on this subject is reprinted in full, in which many instances of cases of typhoid occurring among the "highly" vaccinated troops after they left the strict-control of the cantonments in the U. S. are noted.

For instance, a replacement unit of 248 men reached England with 98 cases of typhoid and the case death. rate was 8.42 per cent. Investigation indicated contaminated drinking water obtained "en route" in the U. S. The unit had been vaccinated a few months prior to the occurrence of the epidemic.

Again it says:

"Following the offensive in the Argonne sector, typhoid and paratyphoid began to be reported from practically all divisions engaged in that offensive. . . . More than 300 cases were attributable to the Argonne offensive. . . . 874 cases of typhoid and paratyphoid reported in A. E. F. since October 1st, 1918" (to about January 1st, 1919?).

If typhoid is prevented by vaccination it ought to work just as well on a battlefield as in a cantonment, but if sanitation is solely responsible for reducing typhoid as the present writer believes, then we would expect such occurrences as quoted above to happen.

However, we find in that "germ-swatter's" bible:—
The Journal of the American Medical Association, for July

28, 1917, Vol. 69, pg. 267, under the heading "Vaccination in War":

Bernard and Paref, in an analytic study, reported in 1915 a great preponderance of paratyphoid infections in the anti-typhoid vaccinated over those in the non-vaccinated, presenting the remarkable figures given in Table 2.

Table 2. Preponderance of Paratyphoid Infections Over Typhoid.

	Cases	Vac-cinated	Non-vac-cinated
Typhoid (Eberth bacillus)	77	45	32
Paratyphoid	248	222	26

Unfortunately, these authors do not give the relative proportion of the normal contingents who were given the antityphoid vaccination. Rest, however, in 1916 reported a careful analytic study of a small series of 215 cases of typhoid infection with 621 controls of non-typhoid diseases, among which he determined the percentage of antityphoid vaccinations.

He finds that the percentage of protection afforded against infection with typhoid is offset by the same percentage of increase in paratyphoid. This percentage is identical to within a figure in the second decimal place.

Labbe also reports in 1916 the figures concerning antityphoid vaccination given in Table 3.

Table 3. Protection Afforded by Antityphoid Vaccination.

	Cases	Vac-cinated	Non-vac-cinated
Typhoid (Eberth bacillus)	241	19	222
Paratyphoid	150	120	40

These French experiences together with those of the expeditionary force at the Dardanelles have shown the relative futility of vaccinating with the simple typhoid vaccine, and have resulted in the serious consideration, and to some degree, adoption by the French of a triple vaccination, simultaneously administered, or of a triple mixed vaccine.

Experimentation by Widal and others has shown that vaccination of animals with equal parts of three heated vaccine viruses (typhoid, paratyphoid A and paratyphoid B) produces . . . evidences of simultaneous immunization against the three infections.

Widal and Courmont regard paratyphoid among the troops as the most prominent epidemiologic fact of the war.

There is an admission in black and white in the most prominent, leading REGULAR Allopathic medical journal, that vaccination, in the cases examined, and in the Dardanelles expedition, in stopping typhoid, has merely substituted paratyphoid for the same, *the percentage being identical to the second decimal place.*

Could anyone but an Allopath look at such figures and still believe in vaccination? *One vaccine merely substitutes a 2nd disease, which in turn is only slightly different from the 1st disease* so slightly that only an allopath is competent to "diagnose" the case. Two vaccines seem to produce a third, slightly different disease, and so EUREKA they will use a triple vaccine which prevents all three diseases. And then came Influenza and Pneumonia.

Now we have already seen in the quotations from several encyclopædias (see earlier part of chapter) that germs do not cause disease, it is the toxins that cause the disease, and the germ merely gives the disease its *"characteristics,"* in other words, all diseases are due to toxins and the "characteristics" or symptoms given by the germ merely indicate to an expert diagnostician which disease is present, or rather which germ is present.

If germs are scavengers as the present writer claims, this would be just what should happen—either the vaccination so modifies the characteristics of these germs that they appear to be entirely different germs, to one diagnosing the case; or else vaccination bars one kind of germ, only to allow another, with different "characteristics," to "raid" the accumulation of toxins, within the body, at a later period.

This appears to the writer to be exactly the condition which brought on our great influenza-pneumonia epidemic. He believes vaccination merely substituted the influenza germ for that of typhoid or that they are substantially the same germ with its "characteristics" modified so as to be diagnosed as influenza by the allopathic physicians.

For instance, in the U. S. Public Health Report for March 28, 1919, Vol. 34, page 614, in discussing the occurrence of typhoid in the A. E. F., it quotes the Surgeon-General of the A. E. F., as saying in part, in a circular on the subject:

"The distinction between mild typhoid, paratyphoid A and paratyphoid B can be made definitely only by the isolation of the infecting organism from cultures of the blood, urine or stools.

"5. Differential Diagnoses—Influenza: Many cases originally diagnosed as influenza in the A. E. F. have subsequently proven to be typhoid. The symptoms which the two diseases have in common are continuous fever without localizing symptoms and slow pulse associated with absence of leucocytosis, etc., etc." . . .Intestinal types of supposed influenza should always be considered as possible typhoid until proven otherwise.

According to the Scientific American for September 20, 1919, the deaths in the U. S. Army during the late war up to March 10, 1919, were classified as follows:

Died in battle..................	48,909	43%
Died of Pneumonia, about.......	47,500	42.6%
Died of Meningitis, about........	2,300	2.1%
Died of Tuberculosis, about......	1,300	1.2%
Died of other diseases...........	5,900	5.1%
Total, died of disease...........	56,991	51%
Other deaths...................	6,522	6%

Total number of deaths to Mar.
10, 1919.................... 112,422

This article shows that pneumonia with which is classed influenza, killed 83.6 per cent of all those who died of disease, while in the Spanish-American war it says typhoid caused 85 per cent of all deaths.

Surely this does not go very far towards proving that

vaccination did much in reducing the actual death rate
from disease in this war, in fact, the same article quoted
in the Scientific American shows conclusively that the final
death rate from disease was only slightly lower than it was
in the Spanish-American war, an amount that could be
more than accounted for by improved sanitary conditions
in the large cantonments, over those that prevailed in the
tent camps of the prior war.

According to Dr. Creighton "300,000 vaccinated and
re-vaccinated persons died from smallpox in India 1884-
1888."

Dr. M. R. Leverson, M. D., in a lecture at Claridge
Hotel in London on May 25th, 1911, in discussing
"The Germ Theory Fetish" said in part. Now, the forcing
of these inoculations upon individuals by law *is one of the
worst of tyrannies imaginable*, and should be resisted, even to
the death of the official who is enforcing it. . . . The en·
tire fabric of the germ theory of disease rests upon assump-
tions which not only have not been proved, but which are
incapable of proof, and many of them can be proved to be the
reverse of truth.

LATE NEWS BULLETINS

CHICAGO SOLDIER GETS LONG SENTENCE.

Chi. D. News.
11-15-'18.   [*By The Associated Press.*]

Camp Grant, Ill., Nov. 15.—Morris Tinsky, a Chicago soldier at Camp
Grant has been sentenced to twenty-five years in the disciplinary bar-
racks at Fort Leavenworth for refusing to be innoculated against
typhoid. Tinsky was a member of company 6, 161st depot brigade.

Dr. A. A. Erz, N. D., E. C., in "The Medical Question" (pg. 220) quotes Dr. W. Hitchmann, formerly a public vaccinator of Liverpool, England, as saying:
"I have seen hundreds of children killed by vaccination.
I affirm that now, as for 30 years past, within my own per-

sonal experience and observation, vaccination has proved itself a curse rather than a blessing, causing, primarily or secondarily, more deaths than any other diseases of childhood. —Smallpox, I repeat, when compared with constitutional syphilis as propagated by vaccination, is like the sweetest and loveliest blossom that was ever washed with morning dew."

Dr. Erz also quotes (pg. 219) a recently published British work entitled "History of the Reign of Queen Victoria," as saying:

"Official statistics prove that 26,000 were annually slaughtered by the poisoned lancelets of public vaccinators and more than 100,000 injured annually by invaccinated diseases."

further on he also says:

Dr. J. Collins, F. R. S. C., Public Vaccinator of London,

TYPHOID IN ARMY IN FRANCE; 132 NEW CASES SET RECORD

WASHINGTON, D. C., Feb.. 26.— Illness amoi.. the American expeditionary forces showed considerable increase during the week ending Feb. 6. There were 132 new cases of typhoid fever, setting a new high rate for this disease.

The statistical review made public today gave the total number of sick reported on Feb. 6 as 79,069, of whom 59,325 were being treateu for disease and the remainder for injuries.

The total number of sick and injured returned from France from the beginning of the war up to Feb. 14 was placed at 69,574, of whom 59,456 had been sent home since the armistice was signed.

Health conditions in the army at home were reported as satisfactory for the week of Feb. 14, with the pneumonia rate steadily decreasing.

resigned, writing "Were I to describe a tithe of the ruin wrought, your blood would stand still. Vaccination transmits filthy and dangerous diseases without offering any protection whatever."

and he quotes hundreds of similar statements by competent authorities.

Now as to the odorless condition of the excrement; of what importance is this or what does it indicate?

The present writer believes that it indicates that all the food eaten has been completely burned or oxidized in the body, and that, therefore, there is no surplus food in the system to putrefy, ferment or decay and form toxins or, in other words, that the excrement is totally free from toxins when perfectly odorless, and hence would not support germ life in this condition if germs are scavengers for these toxins. This would account for the writer's apparent immunity to germ action while his excrement is odorless.

However, the allopathic fraternity doesn't consider the condition of the excreta of any consequence apparently, as they (or many of them) will sit by and say that nothing can be done to save a sick man, without making any effort to examine the excreta, and only sneer at the idea that enemas might be of any use, although it would only cost about 1 cent a day to try them.

The allopath's stand is probably based on the belief that germs and nothing else cause disease and, of course, if this were true, enemas would not be of much use. Their opinion of the importance of odorless excreta is probably truly represented by the statement made by Williams & Williams in "Laboratory Methods," 3rd Ed., p. 149, where in describing the examination of stools, they say:

"Stools are generally so offensive that their examination in private practice is often discouraging and is never necessary as a routine procedure.

Odor.—This is of little diagnostic import. There may be little or no odor in starvation and certain chronic diseases, but the odor of a meat diet is most marked......

"*Searching for Bacteria.*—As a routine procedure, this is of little practical value because of the enormous numbers and varieties of germs normally present.".....

Value and Limitation of Stool Analysis.—"A routine stool examination in every case of sickness is worse than a waste of time to the physician."

To this the present writer must say that he believes

there is nothing which will give such a true and exact indication of the amount of toxic material in the bowels as the odor of the excrement.

An engineer would never think of judging the efficiency of a boiler plant without at least a rough estimate of the unburned coal in the ashes and partly burned gases going up the stack, but an allopath apparently doesn't even know that a foul odor of the excreta is an indication of undigested food that can't be entirely burned or oxidized by the body, hence an "examination" is worse than a waste of time, to him, at least.

Mr. Horace Fletcher says in "The A. B. Z. of Our Own Nutrition" (p. 10) discussing the "Digestion Ash":

What It Should Be Like When It Is Normal.

First:—In adults, or in children after the eruption of teeth and the ingestion of solid food: The non-liquid and non-gaseous waste of the human body *which, in its normal state, is not offensive*, should be very small, in quantity, should be pillular in form, either separate or massed together; should have no odour when released, should take on no odour on standing, should be entirely aseptic (non-poisonous); should drop freely from the exit, leaving nothing behind to wash or wipe away. It *may* not be collected in the intestines of full grown and elderly persons, when normal, as above, in sufficient quantity to require or necessitate emptying oftener than from twice a week to once in two weeks; according to age, activity, etc. . . .

Second:—Economic Digestion-Ash (solid excreta), as a daily average for an adult of 140 lbs., (63.5 kilos.) including moisture, when released should not weigh more than two ounces (56.70 grams), an average of less than one-half this amount of waste has been secured in test experiments.

Third:—The true test of healthy Z (excreta) *is absence of odour and completeness, ease and cleanliness of delivery.* Frequency or otherwise does not so much matter. Quantity, too, is not so important, but with foul odour there is disturbance, strain and danger.

The normal man is a cleanly being with all excreta in-

offensive; and by these tokens he may be his own private judge. . . .

This curse of putrid excreta caused more deaths from enteric fever during the Boer War in South Africa than all other causes. It is equally a menace to the health and even to life while being formed and carried in the body.

Fourth:—Offensive excreta are quite certain evidence of neglect of the self-controllable parts of our nutrition. They are the tell-tale condemnation of ignorance or carelessness. Each person should learn to read the true bulletins of his health conditions in his waste-products of digestion. Z is the form the body must assume to render emptying of the digestion-ash natural and easy. Man was built to squat on his heels in defecating, and sitting erect on a modern seat is like trying to force a semi-solid through kinked hose. *Healthy human excreta are no more offensive than moist clay and have no more odour than a hot biscuit.*

Surely here is a most remarkable difference of opinion. Williams & Williams book is marked as being copyrighted and published in 1915, while Fletcher's book was copyrighted and published in 1903, twelve years earlier; haven't the allopaths heard of Fletcher's book yet, or does the fact that he does not have an allopathic diploma place it outside the pale of approved literature, or has the allopathic profession's bungling methods of trying out his ideas given them the black eye?

Dr. J. H. Kellogg in "The Stomach" (pub. 1896) ascribes the

"gradual deterioration of the organism by which the tissue-modifications characteristic of old age are brought about"

to these toxins and poisonous ptomains circulating in the system, which toxins, of course, he ascribes in turn to germ action.

Now if these toxins caused old age, removing the toxins and keeping the body entirely free from them should give eternal youth, should it not?

Fisher and Fisk in "How to Live," p. 81, say:

IMMORTAL ANIMAL CELLS.

"So far as science can reveal, there seems to be no princip' limitating life. There are many good and bad reasons why men die, BUT NO UNDERLYING NECESSARY REASON WHY THEY MUST DIE. The brilliant Carrel has kept tissue cells of animals alive outside of the body for the past three years. These cells are multiplying and growing, apparently unchanged by time, to all appearances, immortal so long as they are periodically washed of poison and nourished in a proper medium. IF WE COULD AT INTERVALS THOROUGHLY WASH MAN FREE OF HIS POISONS AND NOURISH HIM THERE SEEMS TO BE NO REASON WHY HE SHOULD NOT LIVE INDEFINITELY."

Now this condition "washed free of his poisons" is exactly what has been claimed for fasting **WHEN CONTINUED TO NATURAL HUNGER** by such authorities as Drs. Dewey, Densmore, Eales, Hazzard, Haskell, Walters and Mr. H. Carrington, for the past 10 to 30 years. It also seems to be exactly the condition of the writer at the end of each of his longer fasts. He can always get into such condition by a long fast that his excreta will be perfectly odorless, breath sweet, tongue clear, apparently immune to germ action as manifested in mosquito bites and other means of infection and as far as he can determine himself, entirely free of toxins.

These statements of Fletcher, and Fisher and Fisk, put an altogether different light on the subject of the examination and condition and odor of the excrement than those of Drs. Williams and Williams, although Fisher and Fisk's book was also published in 1915, hence it cannot be claimed to be much later authority.

In this possibility of living indefinitely, if you can wash yourself free of toxins, lies the real importance of fasting to natural hunger, as the writer's experience clearly proves that this result can be attained in this manner, pro-

vided you fast long enough, and, of course, take plenty of
nemas to keep the bowels empty throughout the fast
(about 20 to 30 quarts a day).

The condition of toxicity of the excrement is a direct
index to the amount of toxins within the body, as practically all toxic material in the body must be eliminated
through the bowels, hence odorless excrement means that
the system is practically free of toxins—and still, the allopaths cling to the belief that examining the condition of
the excreta "is worse than a waste of time."

The Bible says:

"Fast ye not and ye cannot enter the kingdom of
heaven."

Could not this mean that eternal life (on this earth)
is obtainable, but only through fasting, and in no other
manner? The writer believes that this may be what it
means. It is said that Fasts help develop spiritual powers.

He also believes the story of Eve's temptation with the
apple is probably a parable to the effect that man's first
sin is overeating, all other sins are an outgrowth of this one.

This belief is strongly supported by an article on
catarrh in the 9th edition of Encyclopedia Britannica where
after giving overeating as the principal cause of catarrh
(although it also erroneously gives other causes, such as
undereating), it goes on to say that "catarrh may lead to
any degree of degeneracy whatever." Now if catarrh is
curable by a long fast, could not "any degree of degeneracy"
that might be due to it also be cured at the same time?

This is indicated by the writer's experience. He has
found that catarrh of the bowels is often accompanied by
unnatural sexual desires, which always leave with the cure
of the catarrhal condition at the end of a long fast.

The writer believes that this condition of life in which
we eat the absolute minimum of food, and keep the excreta

perfectly odorless at all times, will bring us to the old Gar
den of Eden conditions referred to in the Bible and greatl
prolonged, or possibly eternal life on this earth—*if* we can
find and stick to the proper diet and manner of living.

Another indication that cleaning the system of the
four poisons that usually are found in the bowels is beneficial to health, is found in a recent article in Physical Culture for March, 1919, where the statement is made that
209 drugless doctors treating 14,841 cases of influenza during the 1918 epidemic, had only 18 deaths, which figures
1 death in 825 cases. The Palmer School of Chiropractics
claims that all of their practitioners had an average death
rate of influenza of 1 death in 886 cases. While the Osteopathic Physician, an authoritative publication, claims that
the osteopathic losses from influenza were only .78 of 1 per
cent.

Now the death rate from influenza during the six weeks
at the height of the 1918 epidemic in Chicago, was 4,825
deaths in 33,968 cases (Tables 9 and 10 of "A Report on
an Epidemic of Influenza in the City of Chicago in the Fall
of 1918," by John Dill Robertson, M. D., Commissioner of
Health) or 1 death for each 7.04 cases or 14¼ per cent.
This includes all schools of medicine, and the writer was
told by Dr. Robertson, Commissioner of Health, that the
records of the office did not show, and were not in such
shape that the death rate of the different schools of medicine could be dug out. This same report (same tables)
gives the death rate of pneumonia for the same six weeks
as 2,842 deaths in 9,748 cases or 1 death to 3.43 cases, or
over 29 per cent.

Don't these both seem to be an extremely heavy death
rate when compared to the drugless doctors' record, and
also when you consider that Fisher and Fisk say death is
not necessary?

The writer believes the principal reason for the great difference in these figures is the neglect of the enema and the feeding and drugging methods of the allopaths on one hand and the use of the enema, fasting and other means of cleaning the system by the drugless doctors.

Bernarr MacFadden and F. Oswald, A. M., M. D., say in "Fasting Hydropathy and Exercise" (published in 1903) (p. 53) that "Influenza (La Grippe) can be nipped in the bud by a few days total abstinence."

The present writer believes that all lung diseases from catarrh and plain colds to pneumonia and consumption, are merely an effort of the body to throw off through the lungs decayed material or body refuse that should naturally be eliminated through the bowels, but because of these being clogged by prolonged overloading, the body makes a last desperate effort to eliminate these poisons through whatever other route is available, and as the blood naturally flows to the lungs for oxygen after supposedly depositing all its refuse material in the natural organs of elimination, it would naturally carry poisons along if it was unable to clear itself of them because of the foulness of the bowels.

During the influenza epidemic last year the writer noticed two articles in the newspapers that would support this view, one was to the effect that 2,000 cases of pneumonia in the army laid out on cots in the open air, or in tents for some days at Brest, France, with insufficient doctors, *and strange to relate, nobody died.* The other article described the experiments of a regular allopathic doctor with serum, and it said that 36 per cent of the cases got well. Isn't that wonderful? Might we be allowed to inquire as to what became of the 64 per cent not mentioned? This certainly looks as though putting these cases outdoors in dog tents was very much better than vaccinating them, at least.

Furthermore, he has heard of four doctors in Chicago,

including two Osteopathic and two Allopathic physicians, all of whom believe in cleaning the bowels out, and whose claims altogether are, that the four of them, in treating over 1,500 cases of influenza, HAVE HAD NO DEATHS WHATEVER; *while nearby are two of the old-time "germ-swatting" Allopaths who had forty deaths in a short time, and in a comparatively small number of cases,* although the exact number of cases could not be determined. The writer believes such statistics of the different schools of medicine for a year or two would soon indicate which treatments should be widely adopted and which ones dropped.

Another disease that needs the immediate attention of the public to the terrible death rate is that of tuberculosis, both pulmonary and other forms, in which the case mortality rate is now generally from 50 to 70—think of it, 50 to 70 per cent of every one who gets this disease dies. Could anything show more eloquently than this that the disease is not being properly treated? If death is not necessary as Fisher and Fisk claim, and 70 per cent of all these sufferers die, it seems to the writer that the methods of treatment being followed should be looked into by a grand jury at once, just as much as any engineer who had 70 per cent of his buildings fall down. Dr. Hazzard recommends fasting and enemas for this disease, while the allopaths overfeed and overdrug the cases and say "the condition of the excreta is of no importance," while they chase that "will-o-the-wisp" the germ theory.

On this point Dr. Robt. Walter says in The Exact Science of Health:

"No process of treatment ever invented fulfills so many indications for the restoration of health as does fasting. It is nature's own primal process, her first requirement in nearly all cases. As a means of promoting circulation, improving nutrition, facilitating excretion, recuperating vital power and restoring vital vigor it has no competitor. . . . Food if not built into structure floats in the blood as half vitalized material in just the form suited to feed bacteria (germs), all the while obstructing the circulation, preventing nutrition and exhausting power. *Feeding in germ diseases, where there is no appetite or power of appropriation, is one of the most destructive methods of treatment ever employed.* It is the process of feeding and developing germs; it cannot feed or vitalize the patients."

The present writer believes the correct treatment for all lung diseases starts with giving one or more, three or four-quart enemas every three or four hours to keep the bowels empty, thus reducing the poisons carried to the lungs, next, place the patient outdoors or by an open window where he will get plenty of fresh air, or in extreme cases furnish pure oxygen to assist in clearing the lungs in addition to the enemas. In this case, however, care must be taken that no ozone is produced in drawing the oxygen from high pressure tanks, as ozone will destroy body tissue as rapidly as it will impurities clinging to the tissue.

If the writer remembers correctly, Dr. Osler was quoted years ago as saying of patients who had Bright's Disease or Diabetes that—

"they generally got along all right until they went to a Doctor and then they up and died,"

while nowadays they treat these diseases by fasting and, although their methods are extremely crude and incomplete when compared with Dr. Hazzard's systematic methods they get such quick cures as to call them "absolutely astonishing."

There are too many diseases, such as Spinal Meningitis, Apoplexy, Heart Diseases, Tuberculosis, Pneumonia, etc., where the Allopaths are practically helpless, and are now beginning to admit that they neither understand the cause nor how to cure these cases, yet, if any outsiders claim to have a cure they will all rush to put him in jail as a quack. Their theory is, that if a "regular" physician

can't cure them, it can't be done, and in the meantime they
are so surrounded with license laws forbidding any one to
treat disease "with or without drugs" unless licensed to use,
believe, and follow their methods, that they are practically
blocking further progress in the discovery of cures for diseases which they admit they can't cure themselves.

In Physical Culture Magazine for October, 1919, Mr.
Melville Durant quotes Dr. Ely J. Jones, M. D., as saying
in the Medical Summary for August, 1919, that if we had
no doctors at all the death rate would only be about 7 per
cent, hence the writer has compiled the following tables to
show what it is *with* them:

A TABLE GIVING THE TOTALS OF ALL CASES REPORTED
AND ALL DEATHS FROM CERTAIN DISEASES RE-
PORTED, WITH CASE MORTALITY RATE (OR NUMBER
OF DEATHS PER 100 CASES). Compiled from tables cov-
ering notifiable diseases reported in 36 states and Hawaii
and Porto Rico, given in U. S. Public Health Report for
Feb. 21, 1919. V. 34, No. 8.

Important Causes	Compiled from Tables on page	Number Total No. cases Reported for 1917	Total No. Deaths Reported for 1917	Deaths per 100 Cases 1917
Rabies in Man	321	30	43	....
Anthrax	373-4	202	62	30.75
Cerebrospinal Meningitis	324-5	4,862	3,241	66.7
Diphtheria	326-7	114,832	11,832	10.32
Malaria, including Mississippi*	328-9	163.306	4·885	2.98
Malaria, not including Mississippi	328-9	22,619	3,886	17.18
Poliomyelitis (Infantile Paralysis)	332-3	4,124	1,535	37.12
Rocky Mountain Spotted Fever	334	56	32	57
Septic Sore Throat	335	1,860	176	9.47
Tuberculosis (Pulmonary)	340-1	88,114	42,569	62.61
Tuberculosis (all forms)	342-3	124,147	91,786	73.85
Typhoid Fever	344-5	53,417	10,082	18.89
Typhoid Fever, less N. D. and Vir.	344-5	49,759	10,082	21.2
Typhus Fever	346	58	20	34.5

*Mississippi reported 140,687 cases and 999 deaths from
Malaria, indicating that the Malaria germ must be the most
widely distributed germ there and probably the one generally
present in ordinary colds.

In the above report the high death rate in some cases
, explained by many such causes as "failure to report
cases" and the present writer does not know to what extent
this may be true, but assumes the great majority of doctors
obey the law as to reporting such cases.

DEPARTMENT OF HEALTH, CHICAGO—YEARLY REPORT
MORBIDITY AND MORTALITY

Important Causes	1917			1918		
	Cases	Deaths	Case Mortality Rate	Cases	Deaths	Case Mortality Rate
Typhoid Fever.....	270	37	13¾ %	347	43	12.4 %
Small Pox	266	4	....	292	2	....
Measles	2,663	62	2.33%	19,620	245	1.25%
Scarlet Fever.......	1,809	46	2.5 %	13,444	624	4.65%
Whooping Cough...	4,345	185	4.3 %	5,156	218	4.2 %
Diphtheria	5,708	723	12.6 %	10,290	1,216	1.18%
Influenza	48,533	6,905	14¼ %	0	201	....
Tetanus	12	14	....	18	23	....
Tuberculosis (all forms)	16,567	3,833	23.4 %	14,908	3,787	25.4 %
Cerebrospinal Fever	224	101	45¼%	354	198	56 %
Infantile Paralysis.	96	27	28.2%	529	187	34.8 %
Pneumonia (all forms)	23,309	6,983	30 %	9,303	5,016	55.2 %
Diarrhea, ententis, under 2 years....	7	2,988	....	20	2,880	....

The writer has compiled these tables to show the
extremely heavy, and, as he believes, entirely useless death
rates now prevailing under treatment that is probably
principally allopathic and which will probably continue
until the allopaths learn that germs don't cause disease and
that drugs don't cure it; and find some method of cleaning
the system, whether they use enemas or not.

As long as we have our health departments controlled
by the "germ swatters" school of medicine, as represented
by the American Medical Association, we will continue to
have these high death rates, partly concealed by combin-
ing their own high death rates with the very low death

rates of the drugless schools of medicine, and further camouflaged by having the number of cases and the num ber of deaths reduced to the number per 1,000 populatioɳ usually where the death rate is heavy; rather than being compared with each other, which would more truly indicate the efficiency of the doctors.

The writer believes Dr. Ely G. Jones was about right in saying we would only have about 7 per cent in deaths if there were no doctors, and that *when the death rate is above this, the treatment received is what is killing the patients rather than the disease.* Look those death rates over again.

He also believes immediate steps should be taken to compel all health officers to so keep their records as to show the death rate or "case mortality rate" of each school of medicine separately, on all diseases and also that the relative case mortality rates be kept for cases in which the bowels were emptied frequently and cases in which this was not done.

Another class of diseases that apparently are not properly handled by the allopaths, are the venereal diseases, such as gonorrhoea and syphilis, etc. They practically admit that these are incurable or are "very apt" to return in a few years, and, although they are always trying some new drug from some "great German scientist," they usually find after a few years' trial that it is useless, when of course the "great scientist" "improves" the old medicine or gets out a new one, and sells it to the same old line of suckers for several years more, and so on, ad infinitum.

Regarding syphilis, Bernarr A. Macfadden and Dr. F. Oswald, A. M., M. D., say in Fasting, Hydropathy and Exercise (published in 1903), p. 55, that—

"A germ disease as virulent as syphilis and long considered too persistent for any but palliative methods of treat-·

ment (by mercury, etc.), was radically cured by the fasting cures, prescribed in the Arabian hospitals of Egypt, at the ime of the French occupation. Avicena already alludes to the efficacy of this specific, which he seems to have employed with similar success against smallpox, and Dr. Robert Bartholow, a stickler for the faith in drugs, admits that it is certainly an eminently rational expedient to relieve the organism of a virus."

Another case of syphilis which was cured by fasting and the milk diet—after 43 shots of "salversan" and a lot of mercury and iodide of potassium had utterly failed to help;—is described in the April, 1921, issue of Physical Culture Magazine.

Regarding the use of these drugs, Dr. Harrison H. Lynn of Buffalo, N. Y., says in the Truth Teller of March 7, '21:

"Syphilis if treated properly according to drugless methods, will never develop into the third stage as it does under allopathic methods."

"Salvarsan—that notorious German product—uses arsenic as its mainstay and there has never been a case of syphilitic blood poison cured by it. . . . though thousands of people have been physically ruined by it."

He also ascribes the development of locomotor ataxia, softening of the brain, shaking palsy, etc., to the use of mercury, though it may take from five to fifteen years for these to develope.

Dr. H. E. Lahn, M. D., says in "Iriodology", that secondary and tertiary syphilis are only mercury poisoning and the symptoms correspond exactly to those found in cases of mercuric industrial poisoning in persons who never had any sexual diseases whatever. He also says gonorrhea is only catarrh of the urethra easily cured on an acid fruit diet and homeopathic remedies.

And yet the country is full of these so-called "Public Health institutes" with long lists of prominent "directors" to lend respectability to, and inspire confidence in the most damnable quackery ever practiced.

CHAPTER IV.

TUMORS AND CANCER

The fact that a small tumorous growth of over twenty years' standing was carried off and completely eliminated during the longest fast taken, caused the writer to believe that tumorous growths of all kinds, including cancer, might be merely the result of overeating, causing deposits of material about the system which the regular organs of elimination were unable to eliminate because of the amount of food eaten, and that a properly conducted fast would eliminate all tumorous growths if carried out to the point where the tongue cleared up, the excreta of the body lost its foul odor, and natural hunger occurred. In fact, Dr. Hazzard mentions a case diagnosed by physicians as cancer of the stomach being cured by a fifty-day fast in her book "Fasting for the Cure of Disease."

In "Air, Food and Exercise" by Dr. Rabagliati a prominent specialist on cancer (page 398) states his belief that

"Overfeeding is the predisposing cause of cancer. The essence of disease is the hypertrophy; the occurrence of parasites the accident. Now the question is what is the chief predisposing cause of the overgrowth? Well what can be the cause except an excess of materials in the blood? And if so, whence came the excess of material which is poured out of the blood in the form of cancerous exudation? What source can there be but the environment of the organism? And of all the facts of environment, what so likely to be the chief cause of the danger in the body as the food?"

Dr. J. H. Kellogg in the "Stomach" (page 278), says in discussing cancer in the stomach that

"Cancer of the stomach is one of the most frequent forms of malignant diseases. The use of alcoholic liquors and chronic indigestion are doubtless predisposing causes of cancer. The disease is greatly aggravated by the use of meat."

Further on page 184 of the same, in discussing "Constipation," he says among other things:

"As a rule, it may be expected that any disturbance in the function of those digestive organs that lie below the stomach are secondary to disease of the stomach. Cancer of the liver is nearly always secondary to disease of the stomach."

The Encyclopedia Britannica, Eleventh Edition, Volume 5, page 176, says in discussing the causes of cancer:

"The very number and variety of hypotheses show that none is established. Most of them attempt to explain the growth, but not the origin of the disease. The hypothesis of a parasitic origin, suggested by recent discoveries in relation to other diseases, has attracted much attention, but the observed phenomena of cancerous growth are not in keeping with those of all known parasitic diseases, and the theory is now somewhat discredited.

On page 175 it says further:

Cancer exists in various forms which although differing from each other in many points, have yet certain common characters to which they owe their special significance.

1. In structure such growths are composed of nucleated cells and free nucleii, together with a milky fluid called cancer juice, all contained within a more or less dense filbrone stroma or frame work.

2. They have no well defined limits, and they involve all textures in their vicinity; while they also tend to spread by the lymphatics and veins, and to cause similar growths in distant parts or organs, called secondary cancerous growths.

3. They are undergoing constant increase and their progress is usually rapid.

4. Pain is a frequent symptom. When present it is generally of a severe and agonizing character, and together with the local effects of the disease and the resulting condition of ill-health or "cachexia" hastens the fatal termination to which all cancerous growths tend.

5. When such growths are removed by the surgeon they are apt to return either at the same or at some other part."

Again in the Ninth edition, volume 4, page 801,

"Cancer is essentially a disease of degeneracy, all statistics going to show its relatively great frequency after middle life; and the mortality according to Dr. Walske, goes on increasing with each decade until the eightieth year."

The literal repetition in the Eleventh edition, Volume 5, page 175 of the larger part of the pathology of cancer from the Ninth Edition, and the admission, Volume 5, page 176, that "our knowledge of the origin of cancer is still in such a tentative state that a detailed account of the theories put forward is not called for" is conclusive evidence that the medical profession has made very little progress in discovering the cause of this disease in spite of all the "organized cancer research" endowed for the work, which has been in existence most of that time and, of course, under control of the allopathic profession. Dr. Kenneth G. Haig says in "Health Through Diet" (page 90):

"The group of diseases caused by food poisoning (in other words Uric Acid) has received at the hands of the profession no generally accepted treatment that really goes to the root of matters. All that has been done consists of the tentative treatment of symptoms, a method that cannot produce permanent improvement, seeing that the cause remains untreated. Therefore, the death rate due to the food-poison group is either unaffected or else slowly increases because the cause remains untreated."

"In order to demonstrate that the death rates due to some of the diseases that are caused by uric acid are increasing on the average, I give a table showing the death rate per million living due to some of the diseases that are caused mainly by errors in feeding.

Death-rate per million living due to	1891	1901	1910
Broncho-Pneumonia		460	490
Cancer	692	842	967
Anaemia	54	59	68
Diabetes	66	91	110
Heart Disease, due to rheumatism....	341	403	480
Apoplexy	908	734	706
Bright's Disease	353	390	389
Suicide	85	96	100

Those who would argue that the diet factor has little

or nothing to do with the causation of the above diseases, I must refer to Dr. Alexander. Haig's standard work, Uric Acid as a factor in the Causation of Diseases, seventh edition, J. F. A. Churchill, London, D. Blackstone & Sons, Phila. A fact that is not without significance is the close connection that the incidence of cancer bears to wealth and the resultant high rate of living combined with excessive tea and stimulant-taking. The richer parishes in London have the highest cancer death-rate. Similarly those towns with the largest proportion of the well-to-do classes have a higher cancer death-rate than the towns with a poorer population. . . . It cannot be denied that in countries where the consumption of meat, tea and beer is small, there the cancer death-rate will be found to be low also."

However, there are other well supported ideas as to the cause of Cancer. Dr. A. A. Erz, N. D., D. C., in "The Medical Question" (pg. 348) quotes Dr. Robert Bell of London, a veteran practitioner, cancer specialist, as declaring it as his belief, after years of observation, that the fearful increase in cancer of late years has been due chiefly to vaccination.

He also quotes Dr. W. B. Clarke of Indianapolis as saying: (in the New York Press of Jan. 26, 1909).

"As Cancer was practically unknown until cowpox vaccination began to be introduced, it is certainly about time to study out the possible connection between the two. Cancer, I believe, is a disease of cell life, a disturbance of its equilibrium, manifested by the rapid growth of cells and the consequent building up of tumor. I have had to do with at least 200 cases of cancer, and I never saw a case of cancer in an unvaccinated person.

"The way vaccination causes cancer is like this: It takes twenty-one years to make a man and but four to make a cow, the former being of slow cell growth and the latter rapid. To put the rapid growing cells, or protoplasm, of a diseased animal (virulently infectious) into the slow growing cells of man—as is done in vaccination, etc., is to disturb the equilibrium of cell life and create that disparity, disarrangement and disorganization which, when the season for cancer comes late in life, results in cancer, if not tuberculosis earlier."

He also quotes Dr. C. E. Page of Boston, Dr. J. J. Clarke (in Transactions of the Pathological Society of London, 1894-95), Dr. Denis Turnbull, M. D., and Dr. Montague R. Leverson, M. D., as expressing very similar views as to the relation of vaccination and cancer.

Dr. Tenison Deane, M. D., of San Francisco, in "The Crime of Vaccination," quotes five cases in which tuberculosis and cancer followed vaccination years later, and wherein only the vaccinated members of the families sickened and died.

Regarding a cure for cancer, Dr. G. L. Howe says in "How to Prevent Sickness" under "Cancer Cures":

"As long as thousands of persons continue to die each year from cancer, there will be a field for quacks and fake cancer 'cures.' Warning is hereby given that *no internal medicine, no marvelous salve, paste or ointment, no fluid injected under the skin or any other similar treatment has ever cured a case of real cancer*, all they can do is to raise false hopes." (The italics are ours.)

Notice that he puts internal medicine, the "Alpha and Omega" of the allopathic treatment, at the head of the list of "never cures."

In "A New Therapeutics" by S. R. Beckwith, M. D. (pub. 1899), discussing cancer (page 218 fol.), he says after discussing the failure of surgery in a number of cases, after some successes,

"This led me to make a careful study of the treatment of cancer in this country and abroad, and I am satisfied that not more than 12% of cancers are successfully treated by removal."

Cancer doctors are located in every part of the country who use chloride of zinc, arsenic, etc., to remove the growth by the destructive effects of these chemicals. This barbarous treatment inflicting severe pain, is not as successful as the knife.

In the New International Year Book, 1915, pg. 121, we find the statement under Cancer, that

"The drug treatment of cancer—chemotherapy—has not realized the hopes which the work of Ehrlict, Wassermann, and others, seemed at first to justify. It is a rare year which does not witness the exploitation of at least one cancer cure."

Again, in the 1918 volume of same, pg. 114, it says:

"From the clinic of Prof. Kronig of Freiberg, as shown by a Swiss medical statistician, comes evidence that as reckoned by a standard of his own, which differs notably from that in common use, that the knife is doing nothing for cancer subjects as a class. He reckons cancer from the day of its first appearance and not from the day on which the patient first seeks treatment. He then compares series of operated and unoperated cases and shows by plotted curves that the extension of life conferred by operation is negligible. Kronig and others convinced by long follow-up investigations that few or no cancer patients are alive ten years after operation, have gone over entirely to the use of radium and X-rays.

". . . The number of books and articles on the non-surgical management of cancer constantly increases. These authors are usually scientific and sensible men who realize the conscientious failure of surgery to cure cancer of the race —however successful with cancer of the individual—and their conclusions are, as a rule, based on biochemical studies which lead automatically to the fact that the disease should be controllable by diet, especially in as far as a reduction in protein consumption is concerned."

These certainly are broad statements to make after all the years the medical tribe has experimented on the long suffering public with internal medicines, surgery, etc. Why not quit drugs and cutting and try fasting for a change. It at least cannot be any worse. No cures from medicine and only one cure from every eight operations is a fine record for people who want to put everybody in jail who differs from them. Is this what the allopaths mean by "regular?" And Fisher and Fisk say death is not necessary if we just wash the system clean. Why not try it?

The present writer considers the regular allopathic physicians as a class, the most incompetent school of doctors in the world today, although they may be generally sincere

in their beliefs. They have no right to accuse of dishonest
motive everybody who differs from them. He believes
it is time they stepped aside and let some one who has been
"brought up on different ideas" tackle Cancer. The use of
Radium and X-rays seems to the writer mere amateurish
puttering which will only put off the day when the real cure
is discovered.

In "Vitality Fasting and Nutrition" (page 611) H.
Carrington in discussing this subject (Cancer) gives other
references supporting this contention that cancer is due
to overeating and should be curable by fasting. He quotes
Drs. Rabagliati, Shew, C. P. Newcombe, Dr. Alex Haig,
and Dr. Robert Bell, as all believing cancer is due to overeating, and as recommending fasting or restriction of the
diet as a cure. He also quotes Dr. Keith as mentioning a
case of a woman who recovered from cancer by living for
two or three years on a small quantity of milk daily (in
"Fads of an Old Physician," page 84). Dr. Keith also
noted a marked relief in all cases when an extremely light
diet was allowed (page 82-3). Upton Sinclair also quotes
Dr. Haskell (in "The Fasting Cure, page 148) as having
already cured several cases of cancer by fasting.

All of these authorities indicate a restricted diet or
fasting as being the best treatment for cancer, and an investigation of their statements will show that they are
founded as are those of Drs. Rabagliati, Kellogg, and K. G.
Haig, hereinbefore quoted, on very logical grounds.

This belief was increased by another case which came
under the writer's observation, a patient who had been a
heavy eater and a heavy meat eater all his life, a strong,
healthy rugged man until he had a stroke of apoplexy when
about fifty-seven years of age, from which he never recovered. The writer tried to induce him to fast for years
to no avail. He would not even restrict his diet as he
thought his ravenous hunger the only true indication as

to what he should eat, and that it should be satisfied. After suffering about eight years from apoplexy, which rendered him almost speechless and very much weakened, he developed an acute case of Hodgkins disease (a disease which according to the Encyclopedia Britannica, Eleventh Edition, Volume 17, page 168, "is characterized by a progressive enlargement of the lymphatic glands all over the body, and generally starts in the glands of the neck").

This progressed rapidly to the point where the swellings on his neck had nearly choked off his breathing. Only by the hardest struggle could he get any air at all. At this point he was finally induced to try a low milk diet—about a quart to a quart and a half a day—but absolutely refused to tolerate enemas at all, on the ground that as his bowels moved every day, there could be nothing to wash out. While he had been growing rapidly worse and was nearly at the point of choking to death when he decided to try this—immediately on starting the milk diet, the swellings on his neck began to go down, so that in ten or twelve days his breathing had returned to normal, although he felt very weak, and was considerably alarmed at this weakness.

Furthermore, the attending physician who called at this time did not believe in the milk diet, nor in fasting, and expressed the opinion that insufficient nourishment was being obtained by the patient.

This effectually ended the milk diet, the patient insisted on eating two or three times a day, and again began to lose ground, dying a few weeks later.

This physician argues that during a fast the good tissue is used up as fast as the bad (poisonous or toxic) tissue, and a person will starve to death before a tumor can be eliminated. But the writer's experience with his catarrh and tumor, and this patient's reduction of the tumors on his neck while on a low milk diet, convinced the writer that such is not the case.

A search through several encyclopædias produced the statement in the Encyclopedia Britannica, Eleventh edition, Volume XIX, page 926, under "Nutrition," that

"During a fast the tissues do not all waste at an equal rate; those which are not essential are utilized at a much greater rate than those which are essential to the maintenance of the organism. For instance it has been shown that during a fast the skeletal muscles may lose over 40% of their weight, whereas an essential organ like the heart loses only some 3%. The essential tissues obtain their nourishment from the less essential, probably by ferment action, a process which has been termed antolysis."

In the International Encyclopedia, first edition, Volume VII, page 474, or second edition, Volume VIII, page 390, under "Fasting," we find

"Abstinence from food may cause a grave condition of the body, and may even endanger life. In an experiment upon an animal which was caused to fast for thirteen days, the more important tissues lost the following percentages of dry solid matter:

The adipose tissues	97 %
The spleen	63.1
The liver	56.6
The muscles	30.2
The blood	17.6
The brain and spinal cord	none

The tissues in general become more watery than in health. As the amount of muscle lost during the fasting period contained about 15.2 grams of nitrogen, more than one-half the lost nitrogen came from metabolism of muscular tissue. In a fasting animal, while urea is excreted and carbonic acid is given off, the expenditure of nitrogen is very small. Glycogen and then fat disappear, and lastly some of the proteid, but as the figures show, the heart and central nervous system are supported and lose but little in weight while other organs are sacrificed to feed them."

Again in Nelson's Encyclopædia, Volume IV, page 582:

"The observations made during the fasts of Succi and others show that the body wastes less rapidly when the patient is kept warm and at rest. The fatty tissues are the first to be used up and later the proteids of the skeletal and intestinal muscles. The heart muscle does not diminish appreciably, and probably it derives its substance from the less essential muscles. In long continued fasts the tissues waste more rapidly during the first few days. Later the body uses its reserves of nourishment more economically."

Furthermore, Dr. E. H. Dewey, the "Pioneer of the Fasting Cure," who was an Acting Assistant Surgeon, U. S. A., in charge of a ward in the Chattanooga Field Hospital in 1864, where, he says in the "True Science of Living," page 30: (The italics are ours.)

Postmortems were the rule in this hospital, and as they were more or less numerous everyone of the hundred days of smoke and flame of Sherman's advance on Atlanta, the opportunity of finding out how little we knew of the variety and extent of diseased structures in our patients while alive was most extensive. When we had a case of pneumonia, of pleurisy, or of typhoid fever die on our hands, it was very generally found that it had been involved with diseased conditions that had given no hint of their existence during life and had without much doubt rendered death inevitable from the beginning. But there was one fact revealed in every postmortem of tremendous significance, that failed to make any impression on my mind other than to remember it. The fact that *no matter how emaciated the body, even if the skeleton condition had been reached, the brain, the heart, the lungs, except themselves diseased, never revealed any loss.*

Further on (page 70) in discussing a very weak case who "could not be fed because there was nausea every day" for thirty-three days, he says that (the italics are ours)

"when death occurs before the skeleton condition is reached it is always due to old age or some form of disease or injury and not to starvation."

This case recovered rapidly upon completion of the fast.

In a later book, "The No Breakfast Plan and the Fasting Cure," Dr. Dewey says:

p. 31 . . . As the months and years went on, it so happened that all my fatalities were of a character as not to involve in the least suggestions of starvation. while the recoveries were a series of demonstrations as clear as anything in mathematics, of evolving strength of all the muscles, of all the senses and faculties, as the disease declined. . . .

p. 32 . . . For years I saw my patients grow into the strength of health without the slightest clue to the mystery, until I chanced to open a new edition of Yeo's Physiology at the page where I found this table of the estimated losses that occur in death after starvation. Fat 97%, Muscle, 30%, Liver, 56%, Spleen, 63, Blood, 17, Nerve-Center, 0%.

And light came as if the sun had suddenly appeared in the zenith at midnight. Instantly I saw in human bodies a vast reserve of predigested food, with the brain in possession of power so to absorb as to maintain structural integrity in the absence of food or power to digest it. This eliminated the brain entirely as an organ that needs to be fed or that can be fed from light diet kitchens in times of acute sickness. Only in this self feeding power of the brain is found the explanation of its functional clearness where bodies have become skeletons.

I could now go into the rooms of the sick with a formula that explained all the mysteries of the maintenance and support of vital power and cure of disease, and that was of practical avail. I now knew that there could be no death from starvation until the body was reduced to the skeleton condition; that, therefore, for structural integrity, for functional clearness, the brain has no need of food when disease has abolished the desire for it.

I could now know that to die of starvation is a matter not of days, but of weeks and months, certainly a period far beyond the average time of recovery from acute disease."

As Dr. Dewey had treated practically all his patients by fasting for twenty or twenty-five years prior to writing the above, and as he was educated as an Allopath and practiced some eleven years before discovering the benefits of fasting, he should be very well qualified to discuss the results of fasting as compared to the allopathic treatment of disease, and his statements being those of a well trained observer should carry a good deal of weight.

Additional evidence that the body has some power of selection between various tissues during a fast is also shown by Case 29, where open running sores later completely healed up without any food whatever being taken.

Furthermore, Aron is reported to have discovered that *the brain and the bones actually grow during a fast,* showing unquestionably that the body can utilize the less important tissues to support the more essential ones.

Victor Pashutin, the director of the Imperial Military Medical Academy, Petrograd, Russia, says in "Pathological Physiology" (a course of General and Experimental Pathology, 1902), part of which has been translated by the Carnegie Institute of Washington Nutrition Laboratory, 1908, in typewritten form (p. 427) that

He has found in his experiments on dogs that when mineral salts are purposely withheld from the animal's food for long periods, other food from which all mineral salts have been removed being given, the animal will use the mineral salts in the body over and over, none being excreted or passed in the urine, as occurs when the animal has a plentiful supply of mineral salts in its food.

Pashutin also records (p. 30 of Mss.), in the cases of hibernating animals, that the growth of granulation tissues on wounds goes on during the deepest slumber, even when every other function seems to have almost ceased and the heart may beat as slow as 1 beat in 5 to 8 minutes, the blood circulation being so slow that cuts made in the flesh bleed very slightly.

Also in Case 18 the statement is made by Pashutin that in the case of a girl of 19 who starved to death because of drinking some sulphuric acid, ruining her digestive tract, that the "dead body was like a skeleton, but mammary glands remained unaffected."

Furthermore, if the writer remembers correctly, Dr. Linda B. Hazzard, a pupil of Dr. Dewey, authoress of "Fasting for the Cure of Disease," and probably the greatest living authority on fasting, is authority for the statement that—

"when a pregnant woman fasts, her tissues. even including such essential ones as the heart and brain, will be utilized as may be necessary to properly nourish the child."

Surely Nature has made all provisions necessary to support and protect life while the body is having a housecleaning, and that this is so in man might be expected when one stops to consider the number of animals such as the horse, dog, etc., which prefer to go without food when indisposed.

Dr. Hazzard wrote the present writer on Nov. 18, 1919, that "in sixteen years' active practice she had fasted nearly 2,500 cases with eighteen deaths, in every case *of death a post mortem never failed to reveal organic* defects which made death the inevitable outcome, fasting or feeding." "I have never turned a patient away," she adds.

This is in the wrter's opinion a much better record than any allopath can show.

CHAPTER V.

LENGTH OF FAST.

Now as to the length of time a person can fast, the writer considers the best indications would be given by a table showing the length of a number of fasts already carried out, and appends a table herewith, compiled from a number of sources, the authority being given in most cases and also a short description and the results where known, although in nearly all cases more complete information can be found by referring to the source quoted.

In compiling this table the author's first idea was to prove by a table of long fasts already carried out that fasting for a long period was comparatively safe, when conducted as recommended by the prior authorities on the subject. Realizing after starting the table that many of the authorities were not easily available to the ordinary reader, even if known to him, it occurred to the writer that a table of fasts should also give an outline of the diseases treated and the results of the fast so that any one who was sick could look up cases similar to their own in symptoms, etc., and be referred to a book where they could probably find a long discussion of the case; as many of these cases are quoted to a length of 10 to 15 pages and a few run to 50 and 60 pages of the authority quoted, hence would furnish a very good description of what to expect during the fast.

The allopathic fraternity have frequently denied that these fasts, such as quoted from Drs. Dewey, Hazzard and others, ever took place because they were not watched by an allopath, but there are so many long fasts that are now quoted on such good authority, that even the allopaths cannot question them; for instance, the 132, 70, 63, and 50-day fasts of men (cases 15, 16 and 17) quoted by Pashutin, and the 117 and 104 day fasts of dogs (cases

60-1), as well as the shorter fasts quoted in the Carnegie Institute Bulletin and the 160-day fast of the hog (case 3) are convincing evidence that these long fasts are possible, and if you admit they are possible, there is no sound reason for doubting that they actually took place, or that it would be comparatively safe to repeat them.

In fact, against the claim of the allopaths that man cannot live more than 2 or 3 weeks without food, we have 7 or 8 different authorities for 23 fasts of over 50 days, 9 fasts of over 75 days, and 1 of 6 months in length.

However, the writer believes that a person will seldom have to fast longer than from 40 to 60 days to allow Nature time to clean out any ordinary diseased condition.

He does not wish to imply that anyone should try to equal these longer records just to see if it can be done. The 96-day fasts of the Cork prisoners should be convincing evidence of that and the writer believes no definite length of fast should be aimed at but a person should be guided by developments in their condition as will be described in Chapter VII.

He also now believes that in persons underweight a complete fast is sometimes undesirable as the body may be seriously weakened by the loss of mineral salts. However, anyone who fears this may avoid it by taking six or eight oranges a day or an equivalent of other juicy fruit, or a pint or two of milk a day (but not over a quart, as this would probably provide more mineral salts than the body required, with the exception of iron). The required salts could also be obtained from Homeopathic physicians or druggists in organic form if desired, but nature's fruits or juicy vegetables are the best source.

SOME NOTABLE FASTS

SOME NOTABLE FASTS

Case No.	Patient's Name and Address Authority	Age	Length of Fast Days	Weight in Lbs.				Water Taken	Objective or Disease Treated	Distress	Results	Remarks
				At Start	At End	Lost Lbs.	%					
1	Guillaume Granet s prisoner at Toulouse. (Am. Ency. VII-842.)		58					Yes		After the first 7 days his sufferings compelled him to take water.	Died 58th day in horrible convulsions.	Tried suicide by starvation to escape death penalty.
2	Capt. Casey. (Am. Ency. Vol. 7, p. 842.)		28					Only a little rain caught.			Recovered.	Afloat in an open boat—no food.
3	A Hog buried in chalk cave. (Am. Ency. Vol. 7. p. 842.)		40	160	40	120	75	Licked damp walls of cave smooth.			Recovered.	Note loss of weight equals 75%.
4	Calvin Morgan. (Am. Ency. Vol. 7. p. 842.)		73					Drank freely.			Was much reduced in weight—recovered.	Fasted account religious motives.
5	A convict quoted by Berard. (N. Int. Ency. 2d Ed., Vol. 8, p. 390)		63					Yes				"Lived on water only."
6	H. S. Tanner, in Minneapolis, 1877. "40 Days Without Food," by R. A. Gunn.	46	42						Low gastric fever, inflamation of the stomach and cardiac rheumatism.	Skin became dry and harsh.	"At end of 10 days was cured of fever" "eyes became clearer" "Seemed to gain in strength" "appetite returned." Decided to see how long he could go without food.	"Dry skin" indicates insufficient water. "No passage from bowels indicates no enemas.

7	H. S. Tanner, in N. Y. 1880. "40 Days Without Food" by R. A. Gunn.	49	40	......	36	None from 3d to 16th day, except 4 ozs. on 10th, then freely.	To prove it could be done. Watched continu- ously.	"Foul breath, nau- sea and vomiting, "slight cere- bral disturbance and mental excitement," "allayed by water."	Appearance indicat- ed intense suffering, 16th day allayed by drinking water free- ly. Temp. remained bet. 97½ and 100- 4/5, until last day when it dropped to 82, indicating food was required.	......
8	"A young married woman. T. S. of L. p. 49.	...	34		...		Typhoid fever. Mental and moral faculties weak, health had always been unstable.	Foul tongue with an intense aversion to food.	"Tongue gradually cleared and was finally cured.	......
9	A young boy. (N. B. P. & F. C. pp. 35-64.)	4	75		...		Drank solution of caustic potash which so burned him that he could not drink water and retain it.	......	He died the 75th day of the fast. Mind clear to last hour, nothing of the body left but bones, ligaments and a thin skin: yet brain had lost neither weight nor functional clear- ness.	......
10	Another child about same age. (N. B. P. & F. C. p. 35.)	......	3 mos.		...		Similar accident.	......	Took three months for brain to exhaust entirely the avail- able tissues. Died.	......

NOTE:—Case No. 8 was Dr. Dewey's first case treated by fasting and it was only because the stomach instantly rejected everything put into it, including water, that it was allowed to go without food. At the end he was very much surprised to find that the body was not any more wasted than it would have been expected of a case that had been fed.

This brought up the recollection that many prior cases which had been allowed to eat as they wished had in some cases eaten exceedingly little. In fact not sufficient to keep up their strength. Studying the facts, he remembered that during civil war days he had noticed, in cases in the army hospitals which died, no loss was ever found in the brain and nervous systems, even though the patient might have been in the skeleton condition when he died.

No. / Case					Liquid taken		Symptoms	Result	Remarks
15 Graxier, a criminal. (Pashutin, p. 684.)	63	Est. 115–120	Est. 52	Est. 55	Seldom took water.	……	……	Died in horrible convulsions on 64th day.	"It indicates that in a man there are no less reserves than in animals." (P. 684.)
16 Youth. (Pashutin, p. 684.)	18	70	……	Est. 50	……	Took spoonful of sulphuric acid.	Could not take any food at all 1st week in urine; vomited. Next four weeks only received little liquid to food, last ten weeks only water, no food.	No albumen or sugar in urine; vomited after every attempt to feed. Lived 3 mos. and 20 days.	……
17 Man. (Pashutin, p. 686.)	48	132	……	……	……	Drank some sulphuric acid.	……	"Starvation appears complete." Died in 4 mos. and 12 days.	Blood 2 days before death contained 4,849,400 red and 7,852 white corpuscles in cu. mm.
18 Girl. (Pashutin, p. 687.)	19	……	……	……	……	Drank some sulphuric acid.	Only complained of thirst.	"Some liquid food was given for 4 mos. but not believed absorbed as it was eliminated too rapidly and no chlorides in urine at all. Last 16 days no food at all." "Dead body was like a skeleton, but mammary glands remained unaffected."	Body temperature began to decrease only at last 8 days of life.
19 A woman. (Pashutin, p. 690.)	47	……	……	……	Water taken.	"Was treated by an ignoramus."	No particular suffering.	After last the course of feeding was spoiled by certain complications and mental derangement set in and she died of exhaustion.	……

No.	Patient's Name and Address Authority	Age	Length of Fast Days	Weight in Lbs. At Start	At End	Lost Lbs. %	Water Taken	Objective or Disease Treated	Distress	Results	Remarks
11	C. C. H. Cowan, Warrenaburg, Ill. (N. B. P. & F. C. p. 117.) (1899.)	....	42	165	135	30	Some, but did not drink much.	Chronic nasal and throat catarrh which would not yield to medical treatment.	Claims he suffered no pains or pangs of hunger.	Complete cure, fasted until hunger returned 42nd day.	....
12	Miss E. Kuensel. (N. B. P. & F. C. pp. 136-143.)	22	45	140	120	20	....	Insane, dropsical	In bed 1st week and part of 2nd.	Tongue cleaned up Hunger returned forty-fifth day. Mental condition cured.	"I did not feel tired or weak but happier and brighter each day of fast" am now well, strong and happy."
13	Leonard Thress. (N. B. P. & F. C. p. 148.)	....	50	209	133	76	....	Violent cold settled on bronchial tubes, dropsy developed. At Xmas '99 Drs. said death was only a matter of a few days.	Craving for food left him after first day.	Cured. Dropsy disappeared in 3 weeks; after 10th day walked 2 or 3 miles nearly every day.	He declares that his ailments have left him and that he never felt healthier and heartier in his life. Took a little orange juice and lemonade during fast.
14	A large man. (N. P. P. & F. C. p. 192.)	65	90	200					Appetite had been abolished by severe throat and bronchial attack.	Dryness of mouth. and such aversion to food and drugs when food as to forbid all eating. Nausea and vomiting was vomited. woes last ten days.	Stomach refused food and drugs when another Dr. was called in toward end everything was vomited. Natural hunger returned 60th day with cure.	The most taxing case Dr. Dewey ever had on account of interference of friends, etc.

Case No.	Patient's Name and Address Authority	Age	Length of Fast Days	At Start	At End	Lost Lbs. %	Water Taken	Objective or Disease Treated	Distress	Results	Remarks
30	Stefano Merlatti. (Paris, 1886.) (Pashutin, p. 742.)	22	50	135	Est. 41	30	Ad libitum a litere 3-4 day, 1st 40 days, much less last 10 days.	...	...	For 50 days fast there were only 3 poor excrements (indicating that no enemas were taken). Heart action normal. Body temp. normal.	Was watched.
25	Geo. E. Davis. (F. for C. D., p. 133.)	61	40 * 10	228	174	54	Enemas daily	Paralysis of entire right side.	Very bad taste all through fast. Enormous quantities of fecal matter removed.	"Complete recovery." "Mentality clear and perfect. Digestive organs perfect." "Pulse, temperature and respiration normal." "Was active."	Broke fast with unfermented grape
24	Maria de Concei-see, of Mendes, Brazil. (Healthology, p. 112.)	17 mos.	6			No great loss in Wt.	...	Epilepsy.	"None."	Recovered.	"Physician found all organs perfect."
23	J. Austin Shaw. "The Best Thing in the World by Mr. Shaw."	45	45	200	175	25	...	Mental and physical powers impaired, eyesight affected, threatened with Bright's Disease.	No weakness.	Gained strength constantly—daily more restful sleep.	...
22	Geo. Prophrter. (Healthology, p. 81.)	52	52	135½	92½	43	...	...	...	Tongue cleared 35th day. Hunger returned 51st day.	...
21	Dr. I. J. Eales. (Healthology.)	31	31	192	162	30	...	Reduction of superfluous flesh.	...	Health improved.	...

*Ate a little for 3 days between.

	Age						Disease	Symptoms during fast	Result	Remarks
26 A. L., Iowa. Male. (F. for C. D., p. 161.)	45	49	......	......	..	......	Digestive derangements.	Not able to leave bed 1st 45 days.	Tongue cleaned 45th day. Hunger and strength returned 45th day. Improvement constant and permanent.	Drs. said chronic dyspepsia.
27 F. N., Wash. Female. (F. for C. D., p. 162.)	41	63	200	140	...	......	Obesity and functional heart disease.	But little faster's chilliness and no unusual symptoms.	Attended home duties and visited author's office daily.	Operation for salpingitis some time before.
28 R. H., Wash. Male. (F. for C. D., p. 163.)	40	50	145	105	40	......	Had a badly congested condition of the stomach and intestines.	No extraordinary symptoms.	Cured. In 2 months afterward weighed 170 lbs.	Drs. called it "Cancer of the stomach."
29 F. O., Wash. Female. (F. for C. D., p. 149.)	46	75	172	142	30	Enemas.	Diffuse psoriasis patches covered one-third of body.	Had faster's chilliness 1st 20 days. No visible improvement until 4th week in exudations and itching.	Cured. Hunger returned.	37 yrs. constant treatment by Drs. had failed to help. "Sores all dried up."
30 L. H., Illinois. Female. (F. for C. D., p. 159.)	32	24	112	......	..	4 enemas daily.	Tuberculosis; examination of sputum showed bacilli; both lungs affected; chills and fever.	Enemas always loaded with bile and old feces to last week of fast.	Periodical examinations showed progressive decrease in bacilli. No bacilli on 22nd day.	General health constantly improved after fast.
31 J. H., Ky. Male. (F. for C. D., p. 160.)	34	35	228	174	54	......	Valvular heart disease. Heart missed 1 beat in every 3.	Excruciating pain until 20th day when passed gall stones. Great chilliness.	Temperature and pulse became normal 20th day. Health finest ever.	Drs. held out no hope of recovery.
32 A. J., Iowa. Female. (F. for C. D., p. 165.)	38	60	285	137	148	..	Bright's Disease, with obesity.	No unusual symptoms.	In 2 months weighed 150 lbs.	Though married 20 years, bore 1st child 1 year after fast.

SOME NOTABLE FASTS—Continued

Case No.	Patient's Name and Address Authority	Age	Length of Fast Days	Weight in Lbs.			Water Taken	Objective or Disease Treated	Distress	Results	Remarks
				At Start	At End	Lost Lbs. %					
33	Van R. Wilcox. (Correct Living by V. R. W., also V. F. & N., p. 220.)		60	......	......		......	Partial paralysis, boils, eczema, kidney disease, constipation, alternating with diarrhœa, rheumatism, hemorrhoids, defective eyesight, baldness.	......	"Completely cured of every infirmity. Wt. before fast 2 yrs. ago 105 lbs., wt. after (now) 160. Muscular development good, growth of hair came in.	Felt so good he walked across U. S. 3600 miles in 167 days on two meals a day.
34	E. P. F. (V.F.& N., p.222.)	...	30	......	......		......	Paralysis.	......	Cured.	......
35	Mrs. R. T. (V.F.& N., p.210.)	32	18	98 Clo'd			Neglected.	Headaches, nausea, loss of appetite. "Pain high on ascending colon thought to be growth."	Pain remained until after 3 mos. of strict dieting.	"Health became excellent." Quite normal except for pain remained 3 mos." "Finally complete cure."	"On her feet and active daily." Fast not complete (to hunger).
36	Richard Fausel, N. D. (F. C., p. 57.)	...	40	385	255	130	......	Obesity and dropsical swelling of the legs.	Hunger 1st week but not afterwards.	"Good."	......
37	Richard Fausel. Second fast. (Mac Fadden's Ency. of Physical Culture, vol. 3, pp. 1283 & 1319.)	...	90	297	227	70	Took juice of 1 lemon daily. 5–6 glasses water daily.	Same.	Rheumatic pains occurred about 50th day followed by nose bleed for about a week.	"Good."	Bowels moved nearly every day 1st 40 days. He walked 15 –20 miles a day and worked every day.
38	Mrs. L. Wallace. Monrovia, Cal. (F. C., p. 64.)	28	30	......	......		......	Appendicitis and peritonitis.	......	"Definitely benefitted." "Perfectly healthy."	4 physicians had failed to help.

No.	Case				Symptoms before fast		"Complete cure."	Diagnosis / Remarks
39	Mrs. C. H. Vosseller, Newark, N.J. (F. C., p. 67.)		19	100	Consumption.		"Complete cure."	Diagnosed by Dr. B. G. as consumption.
40	A young lady, school teacher. (F. C., p. 84.)	8			"Anaemic." "Threatened with Consumption." "Exophthalmic goitre slowly choking her to death." "Colds and headaches."		"Perfect cure." alert bright, and athletic.	"Lives on about 1200 calories a day" (since fast).
41	H. E. Hoover, 1910. Knoxville, Tenn. (F. C., pp. 111-3.)	13		2 enemas daily.	Constipation ten years. Piles and resulting pruritis 8 years, bronchitis and eczema of scalp. Asthma, catarrhal deafness, sore throat, intestinal catarrh and a general neurasthenic condition.	Never too weak not to move around.	"All vanished."	He says: "Spent over $500 in last 10 years trying to get well on medicine." "I am through with drugs."
42	Rev. J. E. Fitch. (F. C., p. 115.)	80	50		"Undertook to outfast Moses."		"Gained in weight toward end of fast." "As vigorous today as he was at 21."	
43	Case 3. Comtesse T. (A. I. & D., p. 59.)	70	4 & 4 & 1		Diabetes returned, copious perspirations. Vision rapidly deteriorated. Sciatica supervened. 250 grms. sugar passed daily.	Marked sensation of weakness.	Sugar entirely disappeared. Sciatica almost left. Health solidly re-established. Eyes greatly improved. Perspiration disappeared entirely.	Cured of diabetes 12 years before by Donkin treatment.

SOME NOTABLE FASTS—Continued

Case No.	Patient's Name and Address Authority	Age	Length of Fast Days	Weight in Lbs.		Lost		Water Taken	Objective or Disease Treated	Distress	Results	Remarks
				At Start	At End	Lbs.	%					
44	M. de W. Case 10. (A. I. & D., p. 70.)	……	3 & 3	……	……	……	……	……	Severe and prolonged attacks of dyspnœa.	……	Marked improvement at once.	……
45	Dr. G. Guelpa. (The author.) Case 14. (A. I. & D., p. 76.)		3 short fasts in 1 month.	……	……	……	……	……	"Photophobie" "Mental capacity reduced — thinking difficult." "Atrophy of will." "Hypermetropia, unable to read over 10 minutes."	……	"Resulting improvement was amazing and was accompanied by an indescribable feeling of well being and happiness. All my troubles departed. I feel 15 years younger."	……
46	A. Levanzin (C. I. Bul. 203, p. 73.)	……	31	*134	104½	29½	21.9	About .95 qt. daily.	Experimental.	……	Recovered.	Eyesight improved 100%.
47	Succi. London, (C. I. Bul. 203, p. 72.)	……	40	*123	92	31	25.3	Yes.	Experimental.	……	Recovered.	……
48	Succi. N. Y. (C. I. Bul. 203, p. 17.)	……	45	147.4	104¾	42.65	29.35	Yes.	Experimental.	……	Recovered.	……
49	Grisoon. 1880 (C. I. Bul. 203, p. 128.)	……	45	……	……	……	……	Not sufficient	Experimental.	……	Recovered.	Blood deteriorated account insufficient water.
50	A dog (Luciani). (C. I. Bul. 203, pp. 78 & 81.)	……	43	*37½	21¼	16¼	43½	Received abt. 1/7 qt. water daily.	Experimental.	……	Recovered.	Kept in a temperature about 65° F.

51	A dog (Awrorow No. 2, (C. I. Bul. 203, p. 78.)	44	*37½	29¼	8¼	22	None.	Experimental.	....	Died (account lack of water.)	....	Temperature dropped last 4 days to 90° F.
52	A dog (Awrorow No. 3, (C. I. Bul. 203, p. 78.)	60	*46½	31½	14½	32	None.	Experimental.	....	Died (account lack of water.)	....	Temperature dropped.
53	A dog (Awrorow No. 4, (C. I. Bul. 203, p. 78).	66	*41½	29½	11½	28.65	None.	Experimental.	....	Died (account lack of water.)	....	....
54	A Dog (Hawk). (C.I.B. 203, p. 78)	117	*58	21½	36½	62.9	Received water daily.	Experimental.	....	Recovered.	....	....
55	A dog (Hawk). (C.I.B. 203, p. 78)	104	*61½	29½	32½	52.5	Received water daily.	Experimental.	....	Died.	....	Same dog as last experiment.

*Figures for these fasts transferred from the metric to English system by the present author.

REFERENCES CITED ARE:—

"Am. Ency." .... American Encyclopedia.

"N. Int. Ency." 2nd Ed... New International Encyclopedia—2nd Ed.

"T. S. of L." .... "True Science of Living," by Dr. E. H. Dewey.

"N. B. P. & F. C." .... "The No Breakfast Plan and Fasting Cure," by Dr. E. H. Dewey.

"Pashutin" .... "Pathological Physiology," by Victor Pashutin, the Director of the Imperial Military Medical Academy, Petrograd, Russia, from typewritten translation by the Carnegie Inst. of Washington. Nutrition laboratories.

"Healthology" .... "Healthology," by Dr. I. I. Eales.

"F. for C. D." .... "Fasting for the Cure of Disease," by Dr. L. B. Hazzard.

"V. F. & N." .... "Vitality Fasting and Nutrition," by Hereward Carrington.

"F. C." .... "Fasting Cure," by Upton Sinclair.

"A. I. & D." .... "Autointoxication and Disintoxication," by Dr. G. Guelpa.

"C. I. Bul. 203" .... Carnegie Institution of Washington, Bulletin No. 203. "A Study of Prolonged Fasting."

CHAPTER VI.

WATER DRINKING, THE ENEMA, LAXATIVES AND BATHING DURING A FAST.

The writer believes a person should drink about 2 quarts of water a day at least, and as much more as he desires. He has found that he feels stronger during a fast if he takes a glass or a half glass of water about every 30 or 40 minutes during the day. He also believes drinking a pint, more or less, a few minutes before taking an enema, tends to supply the body tissues with what pure water is required, hence reducing the amount of the enema water that is absorbed by the system, and in this way reducing the amount of poisons reabsorbed from the intestines.

However, Dr. Dewey advises that the thirst should be the only guide as to the amount of water drunk. He apparently believes that the body will call for whatever is required, and that the resulting thirst should be just satisfied, whether it takes a pint or 4 or 5 quarts of water a day to do it. He contends that if more water is taken than the body actually needs, it will have a tendency to dissolve and carry out mineral salts, etc., which are needed by the body during a fast, and would probably not be lost if a smaller quantity of water were used.

He also believes an unnaturally large thirst is an indication of an unusually heavy requirement for water and should be satisfied.

It seems to the writer that the use of the enema while fasting is very important, if not absolutely necessary, as the bowels generally will not move naturally during a fast and the most important object in fasting is to enable the body to throw off poisons through all channels available. This it cannot do through the bowels, the natural outlet, unless they are kept comparatively free from poisons at all times, as any poisons that accumulate in the bowels very quickly begin to be absorbed by surrounding tissue. When a person has not eaten for several days and has not emptied the bowels in that time, such a mass of fermenting and putrifying material accumulates there that the blood which is bringing impurities to the bowels from all parts of the system, soon finds the bowels so foul that it absorbs more impurities there, instead of leaving what it brought, and carries the whole to some other part of the body, frequently the lungs or kidneys, which may become so overloaded as to break down, causing consumption or kidney trouble; or the brain, causing biliousness or apoplexy; or it may deposit these poisons in some weak part of the body, causing some such tumorous growth as soft tumors or cancer.

In fact, the writer believes this is the manner in which all disease starts and develops, the fact that one is fasting tending to accentuate the generation and absorption of toxins from the bowels and hence requires unusual means to remove these poisons from the bowels as fast as deposited there by the blood.

Dr. Hazzard characterizes enemas as absolutely essential, and the writer's experience would indicate that a very frequent use of the enema does about 60 per cent of the work of cleaning the body, the fast proper merely having two functions: 1st, *stopping pollution* by not adding fresh food every day to decay in the body; and 2nd, increasing elimination by allowing the digestive organs and blood to stop the normal digestive functions and turn all their available energy on the one effort to cleanse the body, and break up and eliminate all decomposing material.

But as the bowels are so weakened by years of overeating, they do not move naturally and hence the body cleansing stops here unless enemas or purgatives are used to keep them empty.

The first thing to be guarded against in using the enema is to keep the temperature somewhat below that of the blood (about 75 to 90 degrees is probably the best) ; as a temperature above that of the blood will so affect the bowels that they will not move naturally again until colder water is used; however, one application of water between 75 to 90 degrees will cure this trouble even after some weeks' use of the warmer water.

Also, as the large quantity of water introduced into the bowel will cause a rapid infusion of the toxic poisons from the bowels to the surrounding tissues, thus inducing headaches, dizziness and other signs of biliousness, it is advisable to use an antiseptic in the water to reduce these poisonous substances as far as possible. There are a number of antiseptics that would give fair satisfaction. Baking soda is quite commonly used for this purpose and is good. Dr. Tilden of Denver recommends that a teaspoonful or two of baking soda dissolved in water be swallowed in cases of fever, indigestion, or fermentation in the stomach (hot stomach) and believe me, it works better than all the poisons the allopathic profession know. This is because most, if not all, feverish conditions in the body follow overeating, and are almost entirely due to an acid condition of the stomach which the baking soda counteracts as far as the quantity taken will permit. It is also so harmless that a considerable quantity can be taken, probably several teaspoonfuls a day regularly for some months would not be injurious in most cases, although it might in some. The writer took probably two to four teaspoonfuls a day for about five years in enemas with no apparent ill effects, and considers it the best for such use as a preventive of toxic infusion from the bowels to the system.

However, Mr. John Maxwell of Chicago believes soda injurious because it is an inorganic substance and he recommends that you make an infusion of one teaspoonful of finely pulverized gum myrrh in one pint of boiling

water, let it stand a few minutes, then strain and add the
clear liquid to five pints of water for a three-quart enema.

In taking the enema Dr. Linda B. Hazzard, probably
the greatest living authority on fasting in the world, recommends that a person get down with their elbows and
knees on the floor, and that 3 or 4 enemas of 3 quarts
each be taken in succession, as rapidly as the prior enema
is evacuated to cause the water to completely flush the
upper bowel. However, the patient will usually find for
the first few days at least, the first pint or quart of water
taken will cause a most forceful and uncontrollable expulsion of excreta before the whole enema can be taken. In
this case the writer generally filled up the bag and repeated
the effort to take a full enema immediately, to reach and
clean out the whole bowel. After the first few days this
premature expulsion will not occur, especially if several
enemas a day are taken at first, and as the bowels become
cleaner the enemas can be held longer until all the material
in the bowel is loosened and brought out.

During the writer's earlier use of the enema, using it
three to four times a day, seemed to bring out three to four
times the normal amount of excreta, most of which was
probably adherent to the inner walls of the bowel, hence
not removed by the ordinary movement of same. But in
the latter stages of the fasting, such frequent use of the
enema would merely result in comparatively clear water
coming out, hence the frequency was reduced to about what
would keep the bowels comparatively empty all the time.

The writer does not use or recommend purgatives or
laxatives of any kind. Apparently most of these are merely
poisonous substances which act to loosen the bowels by exciting the body tissue to break down and give up part of
their combined water to wash out the poison in order to
prevent its absorption by the tissue; and, of course, the
deadliest poison (such as calomel, a mercury compound)

will get the most rapid and forceful effort of the body to throw it off, while the least injurious poisons will produce the slowest action. Where a person cannot obtain or tolerate enemas for any reason, these drugs might be used sparingly for a short time, but the writer would advise that about a quart of water be drunk with the medicine to save the combined, or organized water of the body as much as possible when this is done.

As the bodily efforts to eliminate poisons will work every channel of elimination to its limit, probably, the material eliminated through the pores of the skin will be greatly increased during a fast and will also probably have a very foul odor; hence a soap and warm water bath should be taken at least every morning and night during the fast.

The writer has found that when the conditions within the body are very foul, even this will apparently have very little effect in reducing the offensive odors given off during the first part of a fast, the materials coming out so fast that the skin is only clean a few moments, especially in hot weather.

As stated before the writer believes enemas comprise about 60 per cent of the treatment in fasting, the real object at all times being to *clean out* the system, and the use of enemas in any case of disease is of more importance than the fast itself, hence those who, for any reason at all, fear a fast, can get most of the benefits due to cleaning the system by a liberal use of enemas with baking soda, and adopting a low and toxin free diet such as used at the Battle Creek Sanitarium, and following this course until the *excretia becomes odorless.*

CHAPTER VII.

INDICATIONS OF THE END OF THE FAST.

Now that we have seen authoritative statements that the less important tissues are utilized by the body to nourish itself before more important tissues are attacked, and that many cases of fasting are recorded of 50, 60, 75 days and longer for human beings and of 104, 117 days for dogs and 160 days for a hog, it is very plain that a fast up to 40 or 50 days should be comparatively safe for the ordinary person.

Some people may say that these fasts of dogs and the hog have no bearing on the fasts of human beings, but we find in "Pathological Physiology of Inanition" by Pashutin, St. Petersburg (a typewritten translation of which has been made by F. G. Benedict of the Carnegie Institute of Washington Laboratories and copies deposited 1 in the New York Public Library, New York City, N. Y.; 1 in Carnegie Institute, Nutrition Laboratory; 1 in the John Crerar Library, Chicago; 1 in the Library of the office of the Surgeon General of the Army, Washington, D. C.), the statement:

"It is generally noteworthy that all that is known about starvation of man coincides with that of starving animals. There is therefore a possibility to make conclusions about man by the facts which we get from animals without fear of running into very great errors of deduction."

Right here the present author wishes to say that he believes there is a real difference between fasting and starvation. The term Fasting in his opinion should be confined to the time when an animal or human being is living on the surplus avoirdupois such as fat, or surplus tissue of any kind (as muscles) that practically every one has in his system and which comprises the less essential tissue first utilized by the body during a fast; in other words, he is living on tissue he can spare while *real starvation* in his opinion occurs when the body's *surplus stock* of material of any one or more kinds necessary (such as mineral salts, proteids, etc.) is completely exhausted, and worn out tissue can only be replaced by taking tissue essential some place else; when this latter condition occurs everyone will acknowledge that food must be taken quickly to avoid death.   Therefore, the present author claims that these two conditions—namely *"fasting" and "starvation" are entirely different and distinguishable by several unmistakable signs which almost anyone can tell.*

In fasting there should generally be no hunger after the first four days without food, although the writer's experience indicates that should a meal or even a sandwich be eaten within three days after the fast starts, you will have to count 3 or 4 days from the last mouthful.   But when food is necessary or starvation begins, a natural hunger sets in that will tolerate no interference with getting food, accompanied by unusual strength, making the faster well able to procure food.

Regarding this hunger during the fast in animals Pashutin says (pp. 84-5, typewritten Ms.).

p. 84 . . . Some of the experiments which we will have an opportunity to speak about below led to the conclusion that the desire for food and water is great only at the earliest days of inanition. Manassein, however, mentioned that the animals also at the last period of starvation manifest great thirst.   ·

Again on page 85 he says (quoting from Albitzky in other experiments) :

"at the later days of starvation . . . only violent force by means of a cage or chain attaches (holds) the animal from undertaking to hunt for something edible."

Again while one's temperature will vary considerably during the first part of a fast and one is very liable to chills as when somewhat bilious, the temperature has a very strong tendency to return to normal towards the end of a fast and should be very steady near the close of the fast, but the minute the patient oversteps the bounds of fasting and is starving for the lack of essential materials, then the temperature begins a sudden drop, continuing until death occurs, usually several days later when the temperature may have dropped as much as 30° F. below normal, although death sometimes occurs before the temperature has dropped this low.

In the Am. Ency., Vol. VII, p. 843, it says (quoting Chossate and Brown-Sequerd's experiments) "this authority just quoted says":

"In man as in animals, the immediate cause of death from starvation is a decline in the animal temperature. Death is accelerated by cold, and delayed by the presence of moisture in the atmosphere."

In "40 Days Without Food," by Gunn, describing Dr. Tanner's 40-day fast in New York, it gives the temperature as ranging between 100 4/5 and 97½ generally until the 40th day, when it dropped to 82 within 24 hours, or less.

In "Pathological Physiology of Inanition," p. 746, Pashutin says, after mentioning a 50-day fast of a man in which the body temperature remained normal—

"however, we know from the experiments upon animals that only when the total of body reserves is consumed the body temperature decreases markedly."

Again Pashutin notes (in "Pathological Physiology of Inanition," p. 33) temperatures as low as 5 and 6° C. (about 40 to 45° F.), in hibernating sleep, and says:—

"A decrease of the temperature of the body is a necessary condition that the hibernation could begin."

Again on p. 34 he says, discussing cold awakening the animals:

"The reason of so great sensibility of the hibernating

animals to the action of cold is clearly in view of the fact that these animals at the time of hibernation have a temperature quite close to that at which life is impossible. The lowest temperature which has been observed (in rectum) at the time of hibernation is in a marmots 5° C. (Prunelle) 4-6° C. (Valentine), in flitting mice 4° C (Saissy), in urchin and dormice 3° C (Saissy), in Siberian marmots 2½° R (Barkow) 2° C (Chorwat). Obviously it is sufficient to decrease the temperature of a hibernating animal to 0.°C. to kill it."

H. Carrington gives 76 degrees as the lowest at which life has survived in the human being, but if animals can stand less, why not man?

Most of the experimental fasts upon animals of which records are available show that when the animal died the temperature had been falling from 2 to 6 days, although it had held well up to normal until the last few days of the fast. (See Am. Ency., Vol. VII, p. 842 fol; also Bul. 203 Carnegie Inst. of Washington—"A Study of Prolonged Fasting," charts on pp. 356-7).

The present writer, although he did not know anything about temperature variations during his own fasting and did not take his own temperature at any time during his fasting, believes that this sharp drop of the temperature noticed at the end of most if not all of these fatal cases, and in many cases which like Tanner's were not fatal, really MARKS THE IMPORTANT POINT OF DIVISION BETWEEN FASTING AND STARVATION, *between having surplus material to support life for some time yet and not having sufficient surplus material to support life longer without eating,* and a close watch should be kept for it by noting the temperature every 4 or 6 hours more or less except during sleep.

Another very important indication of the completion of a fast in the writer's opinion, at least when the bowels have been kept properly emptied by mean's of enemas, is that the excreta, which may and does become indescribably offensive in odor during the greater part of the fast; when the toxins and all foul matter are completely eliminated, *becomes PERFECTLY ODORLESS,* this in the writer's case *always* coincided with the return of natural hunger and other signs of the completion of the fast, such as the clearing of the tongue, and these signs were accompanied by an entire elimination of the foul taste in the mouth and very foul breath present during the fast; the taste and .breath becoming very pleasant and sweet and clean. This odorless condition of the excreta as an indication of the completion of the fast is noticed by Hereward Carrington in "Vitality Fasting and Nutrition" and also by Dr. Hazzard in "Fasting for the Cure of Disease."

Again, during a fast, at any time when the patient has been 24 hours without any food, the tongue will be coated in proportion to the impurities in the body, but when natural hunger returns, if the bowels have been properly kept empty, it will gradually clear up some time during the latter part of the fast. It will often clear up immediately on eating a little and remain clear some hours; however, so that it should be judged about 24 hours or more after the last food was taken in case one eats occasionally during his fast.

The breath will also become pure, sweet and clean at the same time the tongue becomes clear and the eyesight will also become very sharp and clear at the end of a fast, practically all authorities have noticed this in a great many cases.

To sum up then, the indications of the end of a fast are:

1st—A sharp drop in temperature below normal only occurring when body reserves are exhausted.

2nd—Natural hunger returns.

3rd—Excreta becomes odorless (if sufficient enemas

have been taken to eliminate all poisons before body exhausts its surplus of tissue).

4th - Coating on tongue will clear up at the same time (before eating).

5th - Taste in mouth changes from foul to very sweet.

6th - Odor of breath becomes clean and sweet.

7th - Eyesight becomes very clear and sharp.

These last four conditions, of course, depend largely on the third and may not occur in cases where the patient finds it necessary to eat because of natural hunger, or a drop of temperature occurring before the poisons are all out of the system.

In this case the proper course would be to continue taking the enemas (and soda) while building the body up on a non-toxic diet, to where another fast could be taken.

CHAPTER VIII.
DANGERS TO BE MET IN FASTING.

In the writer's opinion, by far the greatest danger to be met in fasting is the so-called "failure" of the stomach to function during the latter part of a fast when an attempt is made to feed the patient before "natural hunger" returns.

Reading somewhere of this so-called "failure" of the stomach during long fasts, prevented the writer from fasting to natural hunger for over eight years, with the result that he got practically no permanent benefit from all his fasting; hence, in the fall of 1914, he decided to fast to the finish regardless of the effect on the stomach, and discovered that while there is unquestionably a time during which the stomach *cannot* digest food, during the latter part of a fast, nevertheless, when natural hunger returns, peristaltic action sets in and the stomach acquires strength and energy enough to handle food in small quantities at first, but in a very few hours attains the ability to handle a considerable meal and do it with astonishing rapidity. For instance: the writer found that the bowels moved almost exactly two hours after eating, whether he ate a bag of peanuts and a 5-cent cake of chocolate only, or a full meal; and whether he ate once a day or three times, the bowels moved *two hours* after *each* time he ate, and moved with a forcefulness and energy never before experienced. The food also seemed to be completely oxidized to an odorless condition and in every way the stomach seemed much stronger and digested food with greater speed than ever before.

However, the writer is not the first to note that the stomach recovers its strength with the return of natural hunger, as Dr. Dewey noted this fact in several places in his books; and although he did not fully grasp the cause, he argued that the body was merely laying aside its ordinary or rather unnecessary functions to utilize all available strength in the more important function of elimination.

This idea is also supported by Hereward Carrington in "Fasting, Vitality and Nutrition," who in addition notes that in every long fast which he has investigated he found that the faster also became sexually impotent during the latter part of the fast, but returned to normal condition upon its completion and the return of hunger.

Dr. Dewey notes in cases Nos. 8 and 14 particularly; where the patients were induced to eat by friends or allopathic doctors who were called in, and were absolutely unable to digest the food offered, in fact, vomited everything eaten during this period, but when feeding was stopped and fasting resumed until natural hunger returned they found no such trouble on attempting to eat; in fact, he repeatedly speaks of the excessive hunger experienced by the patients at the end of their fasts and of their enormous capacity for food at this time.

In the present writer's opinion, practically all the deaths of fasting patients which have occurred after the patients have come under control of allopathic physicians, were due solely to this "premature" effort to feed them and not to the fasting, and hence due only to the meddlesome interference of the allopaths. One instance of this is the death of the English woman for which Dr. Hazzard went to jail some few years ago. She did not die while under Dr. Hazzard's control, but after the allopaths had decided that (in their opinion) the fast had gone too far, and had stepped in and either induced or forced the poor woman to take food. This case is strikingly like case 14, mentioned above where one of Dr. Dewey's cases nearly died through the efforts of friends and an allopath to feed him, but finally discharged the allopath and continued the fast to natural hunger, and a successful cure; except that the poor woman failed to get away from the allopathic treatment and undoubtedly died of poisons from the decaying food which she could neither digest nor eliminate in any other way. These poisons are undoubtedly the cause of most of the deaths caused by premature feeding after a long fast.

In the writer's opinion, whenever a patient who is fasting, or his friends think feeding is necessary before natural hunger comes, a stomach pump should be available and the stomach emptied of everything remaining there after 4 or 5 hours have passed since eating, as Borchard says digestion ceases about 5 hours after eating and decomposition sets in in the stomach, even in comparatively healthy people.

However, the writer's experience with this condition clearly indicates that in many cases, at least, the stomach cannot be induced to take food until the system is cleaned out and hunger returns, and he would recommend as Dr. Dewey, Dr. Hazzard and Hereward Carrington do, that all cases of fasting be continued to natural hunger.

On this point Mr. Carrington says in "Vitality, Fasting and Nutrition," page 543:

"I must contend, and that strenuously, that the breaking of the fast prematurely is one of the most foolish and dangerous experiments that can possibly be made * * * (page 544). I wish to impress the following statement upon the minds of my readers, since it is one of the most important facts contained in this entire book; and the failure to appreciate it is, I believe, the cause of almost all the misunderstandings concerning the fasting cure—showing the complete ignorance of the philosophy of this method of treatment.

The statement is this: **Nature will always indicate when the fast should be broken** and there can never be any mistake made by those who are accustomed to watching fasting cases as to when to terminate the fast.

The average death rate or "Case Mortality Rate" of both Dr. Dewey's and Dr. Hazzard's cases, each having treated several thousand cases by fasting, has been only about 1 per cent, including all cases not carried to natural hunger, as well as those that were; but on those cases in which the allopaths have stepped in and induced or forced the patient to eat too soon, the death rate has been much greater, probably nearer 50 per cent. This is one reason that fasting is so thoroughly discredited among the allopathic profession. They seem to think that there is nothing to fasting, but going without food for a short time and no need of reading prior authorities on the subject, as they seem to look on them as either ignoramuses or crooks, hence in almost every case where an allopath is in control of a fast it is too short; also, generally they use no enemas (although Dr. Hazzard characterized enemas as "absolutely essential") and usually insufficient drinking water, hence fail to get any of the results claimed for it by those who understand how to conduct a fast.

The Bible says, "Let not thy neighbor know when thou fasteth," and in the writer's opinion this is the only safe thing to do when "thy neighbor" is an allopath, and will be the only safe course until such time as the allopaths come to recognize that a person can live on their own tissues without injury a much longer time than is required for most ordinary cases of disease to be cured.

Another apparent danger which, however, is only dangerous because of the fear it inspires in the patient, causing or tending to induce him to give up the fasting treatment, is the weakness that often accompanies cases of fasting of persons whose system is permeated with decomposing or toxic material, such as occurs in catarrh of the stomach and bowels, and probably in such cases as apoplexy, tuberculosis, cancer, or, in fact, any serious case of illness.

The writer has been so weak that for weeks at a time his knees seemed ready to give way under him in a few more steps; however, he has always been able to get around at nearly his normal pace, and has covered as much as 25 miles a day while in this condition, feeling considerably fresher and stronger at night than in the morning, probably because from heavy breathing all day an unusually large quantity of oxygen was absorbed.

At the end of long fasts this absorption of more oxygen than usual always seems to occur and greatly increases the strength. It is also undoubtedly largely responsible for the excreta becoming odorless at this time, as the writer has noticed in every fast carried to natural hunger.

Additional proof that this weakness accompanying the fasts of most sick persons is more related to the poisons in the system than to lack of food is indicated by the feats of Prof. Gilman Low of New York City, quoted by Dr. Eales in "Healthology" as having broken several world's lifting records after short fasts and, in fact, completely established the fact that he could do about twice the lifting after short fasts up to 10 days, as he could on three good meals a day.

There has also been a great deal of dispute in the past as to the injurious effect of fasting upon the blood and its "drying-up" effect upon the skin, both seem to have been frequently noted by early investigators in fasting cases and both, the present writer is convinced, are solely due to insufficient drinking water being taken. This seems to have been one of the causes of difficulties which was unsolved, generally because of lack of experience with fasting.

For instance, the Carnegie Institute of Washington, Bul. 203, p. 25, in discussing the effect on the blood of fasting, says:

Curtis (Proc. Am. Ass'n Adv. Science, 1881, 30 pp. 95-105) made systematic observations of Griscom's blood during his 45 days fast in 1880. This constitutes the longest period with blood examinations of which any record could be found.

Curtis describes the morphology of the erythrocytes as follows:

The first examination, made just after Griscom's last meal, showed the cells in abundance, of bright color, regular,

smooth of outline, solid in appearance. and of usual size—
1/3100 inch. *36th day* "Saw an erythrocyte undergo direct division. From this day on the red cells changed for the worse.
They became pale, ragged and shrivelled. At this time the
subject showed signs of weakened circulation—vertigo, numb-
ness of hands and feet. *39th day*. There was scarcely a normal
corpuscle to be seen. *40th day*. After an excursion of 2½
hours on the lake, there was a remarkable· change in the
blood picture The ragged, pale and broken corpuscles all
disappeared and all the erythrocytes became smooth in out·
line and bright in color. They seemed quite normal, except
that they were smaller, averaging 1/3500 inch. After this
they again retrograded, became soft. pale and sticky, but never
so bad as just before the lake excursion. .   .   .

This gradual and continuous deterioration in the
blood might be due to any cause, of course, but the fact
that the blood became "quite normal except smaller" after
being 2½ hours over a lake would, in the absence of other
possible causes, point very clearly to dampness absorbed
through the lungs during this excursion as the cause of
this sudden restoration of the blood. An investigation by
the writer of several other cases also showed that in all
cases in which the blood deteriorated markedly, insuffi·
cient water was taken. while in those in which water was
drunk freely there seemed to be no deterioration in the
blood.

This is somewhat grudgingly admitted in Carnegie
Inst. Bul. 203, page 156-7, where the statement is made
in the chapter on "The Blood" under
          "Discussions and Conclusions."
The results of the above studies are conspicuous rather
from the absence than the presence of striking alterations in
the blood picture.

The final conclusions as to the effects of uncomplicated
starvation on the blood to be drawn from the results of
examinations on Levanzin, are:

---

5. In an otherwise normal individual, whose mental

and physical activities are restricted, the blood as a whole is able to withstand the effects of complete abstinence from food for a period of at least 31 days, without displaying any essentially pathological change.

Another trouble that may be met in fasting is impotence. Mr. Carrington says in "Vitality, Fasting and Nutrition," that he has talked with many persons who had fasted and found that in every case of a long fast the patient became impotent. Mr. Benedict, in the Carnegie Institute Year Book for 1918, the writer believes, speaks of animals which lost their reproductive powers on a mineral salt-free diet. Could there be any connection between these facts? The writer cannot say that impotence during a fast is due to the loss of mineral salts, and to nothing else, but it seems to him that this could easily be the cause. It seems to cling to a person who adopts a diet low in mineral salts after a fast, but to be more easily corrected on changing to natural foods high in minerals, particularly iron and calcium. Iron is found in lettuce, spinach, grapes, raisins, strawberries, etc., and, milk, though very deficient in iron contains considerable calcium, in fact so much that a pint a day would about supply the body's requirements of calcium.

Carrington also says that impotence is generally corrected at the end of a fast, but the present writer has found that this is not always so. Probably this is due to exhaustion of the body resources in minerals or some other source of vital power, as in some cases it takes a considerable time on a natural diet to overcome the condition following a fast.

It is possible that impotence might be avoided by taking daily allowances of fruit juices equivalent to six or eight oranges; alternating at intervals with a pint of milk a day, but it can at least be considered that importance is cureable when it does occur.

For further information on the dangers to be met in fasting the writer would respectfully refer the reader to "Vitality, Fasting and Nutrition," by Hereward Carrington, where a full discussion will be found of most of the difficulties that can be met in fasting, particularly in Chapters V and VI "Physiological Effects," where a discussion of its effects on The Stomach, The Lungs.; Liver and Kidneys, The Bowels, The Heart, Muscles, Blood, Brain and Nervous System. The Sexual Organs, etc.; goes into great detail; and Chapter VII, "Crises and What to Do When They Occur," where "Famine Fever,"—the frequent apparent *increase in intensity* of a disease because of increased elimination when starting a fast,—Fainting Spells, Dizziness, Headaches, Pain in the Heart, Palpitation, Vomiting, etc., etc., are discussed at such length and by an author whose experience with fasting is so much broader than the present author's that there is practically nothing the present author could add, except his most hearty approval of the statements made therein.

Dr. Hazzard's book, "Fasting for the Cure of Disease," also discusses these difficulties more briefly than the above, and the third volume of Macfadden's "Encyclopedia of Physical Culture" has a very good discussion on the subject.

CHAPTER IX.

THE NATURAL DIET FOR MAN.

It has already been noted that the writer's experience led him to believe that man's proper diet is a diet which will give, first, odorless excreta as a first requirement, and second, sufficient nourishment to sustain life and give the required amount of energy.

To meet the first requirement and eat the amount of food recommended by Voit and others of the older authorities on diet, the writer's last five years of dieting has shown to be impossible. Consequently. he believes it necessary to eat very much less than the Voit standard to have the proper diet. Now on what scientific basis does the Voit standard rest? He appears to have watched a group of ordinary men totally ignorant of scientific methods eat what they wanted, and then measured what they ate without any reference to what condition this was in after going through the digestive tract, i. e., without any analysis to see whether or not this food was completely burned or oxidized in the body as it should be. Any engineer in examining the efficiency of a boiler would not only measure the amount of coal and water used, but would also measure the amount of coal that went out in the ashes and flue gases unburned and partly burned, but this part of the examination was omitted by Voit and seems to be omitted by most of the later authorities.

As already noted, Williams & Williams say, "a routine examination of the stools is a waste of time to the general practitioner," and few even think of the material thrown off by the lungs.

Now is it a waste of time? Mr. Horace Fletcher quotes in the "A. B. Z of Our Own Nutrition," an experiment wherein a comparison was made between his own metabolism and another man's, in which Mr. Fletcher gained in

weight on 3/17 of the quantity of solid food eaten by the
other man as shown by the table reproduced herewith from
page 38, and had dry odorless excreta, whereas the other
person had over 10½ times as much excreta with a very
foul odor.   In the writer's opinion, Mr. Fletcher's condi-

Table of two experiments in Metabolism from page 38
of the "A. B.-Z. of Our Own Nutrition," by Horace Fletcher.

	Dr. Snyder's Experiment Published in Bul. 43	Writer's (H. Fletcher's) Experiment
Age of subject	22	30
Duration of experiment	4 1-3 days	5 days
Weight at beginning............	62.5 kilos	57.3 kilos
Weight at end................	62.6 kilos	57.5 kilos
Potatoes (daily average).......	1587.6 grms.	159.4 grms.
Eggs (daily average)	411.08 grms.	124.7 grms.
Milk (daily average)	710 cc.	710 cc.
Cream (daily average)	237 cc.	237 cc.
Daily urine	1108 grms.	1098 grms.
Daily feces	204 grms.	18.9 grms.

Mr. Fletcher's excreta was practically odorless.

tion clearly indicated that he had enough nourishment;
the odorless condition of his excreta indicates that it was
completely oxidized or utilized by the body, while the foul
odor of the other person's excreta is an indication that
the excess of food eaten by the second party was a total
waste of material that in addition had an injurious effect
upon the system through the toxins generated in the body
because of its not being completely oxidized or burned.

Now Dr. Eales in Healthology (p. 40) quotes Dr. A.
Rabagliati of England as saying in "The Functions of Food
in the Body," that

"According to opinions so generally accepted, as that it
may be said to be universally so, the functions or uses which
food subserves in the human body are three. These are:

1. Food must be taken into the body in order to repair the waste which the body sustains in doing or performing work. It must also be taken in order to provide material out of which the growing body is formed. I admit the truth of this proposition in both its forms.

2. Food must, it is said, be taken in order to provide the source or material from which comes the energy of life. The work done by the body comes it is said, from the food. There are, however, two views as to how this comes about. Some think that the work comes from the consumption of the bodily tissues themselves, while others think that food oxidation is the source of the work, without the necessity of its first being converted into body stuff. On both these views, however, the food may be considered as the source of the work of the body because the body is made from the food. On the former view the food is the somewhat remote source of the work-energy of the body; on the latter view the food is the immediate source.

3. The third accepted, or almost universally accepted view as to the functions of food, and the need of taking it into the human body, is that it is said to be the source of the heat of the body. The food is believed to provide the heat by which the body of a warm-blooded human being is maintained at a temperature many degrees higher than that of the air (or water or earth) in or on which he lives.

I am sorry to say that I disagree with the belief, the common scientific belief, in the truth of both of these last two opinions. I am perfectly certain that the food is not the cause of the work of the body, either of its intellectual. moral, emotional, or volitional work on the one hand, or of the mechanical work of the body, whether internal, as in the various manifestations of functional activity, or external, as in locomotion, or the doing of what is commonly called work, on the other. The food has no relation whatever to these things, other than that very indirect one which is connected with the first admitted function of food. namely, the building up of the body structures, so as to fit them to be the means or medium through which energy acts. The body is, in my view, the medium for the reception, storage and transmission of energy, but neither it, nor the food out of which it is made, is the source of the energy. Nextly, I think it is open to very grave question whether the oxidation of food is the cause even of the maintenance of the bodily temperature. The task of this treatise is to put the reader in possession of the evidence which has made me quite certain on the first point and almost so as to the second."

Dr. Eales goes on to say, p. 4 :

"I have always contended that the human body derived its energy otherwise than can be explained by the food ingested and digested. I proved that very conclusively to my *own* mind during my fast, when I possessed the same amount of strength at the end as I had at the beginning of the fast, and as far as temperature was concerned, my temperature was normal the entire period of thirty-one days without food. · Truly the contention of the learned Dr. Rabagliati deserves careful consideration and study before denial. Old theories are fast being dethroned in the light of modern study and research, and of this wonderful body of ours, this temple of the indwelling spirit, are new faculties, functions and capabilities continually being discovered.

Food, then, supplies the necessary elements which are required by the vital force in building, maintaining and repairing the body. But food cannot import more than it contains. Dead food cells cannot make living blood cells, but rather the living cells of the body use the mineral elements of the food to work with the fluids of the living body to build new cells, in connection with the life-giving oxygen— the breath of life—as every cell must contain oxygen. The human body must be likened to a great movable or automatic manufacturing plant with its many complicated animated machines. The *brain* system is the motor that supplies the power, force or energy for operating the various machines and moving the entire plant at will. The *nerves* are the belts that run to the different machines, over which the electric current passes from the brain to operate them. *Food* is the raw material which is first ground and pulverized in the mouth and mixed with dissolving juices, then given to the stomach, where it is further mixed and churned and more juices added to the mixture, which is elaborated, assorted and passed to the blood stream to be conveyed to other organs of elaboration and perfection, thence on in the blood stream throughout the entire body to supply the elements necessary for the repair of the various machines of the body as well as the building or structure which contains these machines. The many different machines, as the heart, lungs, liver, stomach, bowels, kidneys, bladder, pancreas, spleen, blood vessels, etc., all have their parts to perform in preparing this raw material. The *vital force* is the master mechanic, the inherent, indwelling animated power that superintends the entire plant and is ever on the alert for strikes or frictions among the workmen. Every cell of the organism is endowed with life and mind which thinks, eats, works, and reproduces, dies and is taken to the crematory, burned up and cast out of the body to make room for living cells which are being continually produced.

The oxygen of the air breathed and the electric currents generated by the working or friction of the various machines produces the necessary heat to maintain the temperature of the entire plant at 98.6 degrees Fahrenheit.

The motor, the brain system, receives its energy or power while we rest and sleep and not from food, otherwise we would not need sleep, but when tired out could eat more food and thus obtain strength.

The *brain* and *nervous system* may be compared to a storage-battery which is recharged every night and during the day furnishes the power and energy necessary for the performance of manual work and the current to run the entire plant with its animated and complicated machinery. The force, power or energy in a muscle is derived from the brain system and not from the food ingested and digested, otherwise the more food eaten the more power and strength of mind and body. The converse we find to be true, viz: all food eaten, over and above sufficient to repair the body waste, clogs the body and mind and weakens and deprives the brain system.

The present writer most thoroughly agrees with the idea that food does not directly furnish heat and energy to the body, but on the contrary, he believes that indirectly— after being completely digested, absorbed and built into the cell structure of the body, it does furnish not only the replacement material required by the body, but also by oxidation of an additional amount of body tissue not required for repairs, the energy expended in work and the heat radiated by the body in keeping up body temperature.

Consequently, he believes that we have three entirely independent and widely variable quantities to figure in deciding on the correct diet, namely:

1st. *Ordinary maintenance,* or repair of the body, which will depend very largely on the body weight.

2nd. *Support the body temperature* by replacing the amount of heat radiated by the body. This, of course, would depend mostly on the differences of temperature between the body and its surroundings, and in a very much smaller degree upon the body area; for instance, on a hot summer day with the temperature above 98.6 (the temperature of the body) the body would lose no heat by radiation; while in winter, when the temperature was far below freezing, the loss might amount to several thousand calories a day, depending on the temperature, time exposed, amount of clothing, body area, etc.

3rd. *Provide the energy required or expended in work,* which would, of course, depend almost exclusively on the work done. However, the writer believes that this will prove to be a much smaller quantity than most people think, owing to the relatively high efficiency of the body.

He, however, agrees that all food not completely digested and built into the body cells becomes more or less toxic and injurious and clogs the body and mind by means of the poisons generated and absorbed by the blood, hence he believes that to prevent this the excreta should be kept odorless at all times.

The fact that he believed that only the consumption of body tissue could furnish the replacements, heat and energy necessary, led him, after many efforts to find the proper diet, to look up the records of the metabolism of some long fasts on record.

On looking up several fasts, however, he noted that

apparently the temperature of the surroundings of the body from which the heat radiated might be roughly figured was not given, neither was any record kept apparently of the unburned or incompletely oxidized material discharged by the body from which might be figured how much the food might be cut down and still give sufficient food to meet all requirements when completely oxidized as it theoretically should be.

In the 30-day fast of A. Levanzin, described in the Carnegie Institute of Washington, Bul. No. 203, the total energy he lost per 24 hours averages for the last 10 days of the fast 1,341 calories, and for the five days just prior to this period it was only slightly higher. The average heat output for the same period from proteid alone was 204 calories and the consumption of fat for the same period amounted to 1,049 calories, while there was no consumption of carbohydrate food whatever after the 13th day of the fast.

As Mr. Levanzin's average weight for the same period was only about 107½ pounds, these figures would have to be increased about 50 per cent for a man weighing 160 lbs. However, as Mr. Levanzin had very clearly *not* reached natural hunger at the time of breaking off the fast, the figures quoted would hardly be the actual minimum possible under the conditions noted.

Not then realizing the important effect of the widely varying amount of heat radiated by the body at different temperatures of the air, the present writer decided to try a diet of about 1,200 to 1,300 calories a day in 1918, the lowest yet used, thinking on this diet he might maintain odorless excreta and good health, but found that during the hot months his catarrh returned in full force. As all his past experience with fasting had convinced him that there was only one cause for catarrh, and that was overeating of carbohydrates, he began to wonder to what extent he could

be overeating on this amount of food. Furthermore, he
noted that during the greatest heat of summer, when the
thermometer was up around blood temperature (98½°
F.) or higher, he did not seem to want over one-quarter
this amount of food.

It then occurred to him that since 1914 he had had a
return of catarrh practically every summer, but seemed to
become practically free from it during the winter. This
pointed to the temperature of the air as having something
to do with the diet and he noted in a few experiments that
starting with odorless excreta and the temperature of air
between 82 and 87, but having no visible perspiration at
this temperature, if he ate from one to three times a day
he would perspire very freely and feel the heat keenly for
about two hours after eating each meal, after which the
perspiration would cease and he would again feel comfortable until eating again.

This led him to believe that a considerable part of our
food is burned to heat the body only, and if so, it occurred
to him that this portion of our food could be largely or
completely dispensed with during hot weather.

Again referring to the fast of Mr. A. Levanzin (Bul.
203, Carnegie Institute of Washington) we note that of the
total average daily consumption of body tissue of 1,341
calories, over 1,100 calories per day were radiated, or lost
from the body, in the form of heat.

Every engineer knows that heat lost in radiation from
any power producer is waste power, i. e., does not do any
useful work, and it occurred to the writer that this 1,100
calories of heat radiated from the body in April and May,
when the air was apparently somewhere around 70° F., was
simply being burned (oxidized) to keep the body temperature up to 98.6° F., its normal temperature.

A cast iron radiator equal in area to the faster's body
(1.6 sq. meters) held at a temperature of 98.6° F., and

with the surrounding air at 70° F. would radiate about 3.850 calories of heat every 24 hours, while if the air also was at 99° F., of course it *could not* radiate this heat, and in case the surroundings were at 41° F. say, it would radiate about twice as much heat.

Now the writer does not pretend that the body will radiate as much heat as cast iron; it undoubtedly will not, but he does contend that the relative amount of heat radiated follows the same laws as govern a steam radiator—no heat being radiated when the air is warmer than the body and relatively large quantities of heat being radiated when the temperature of the surrounding air is far below body temperature, clothing, of course, acting as insulation.

That the temperature of the body's surroundings is a very vital consideration is also clearly shown by the statement in the Ency. Brit., Vol. 19, p. 926d.

Under "Nutrition"—Factors which influence normal metabolism:

1. "Fasting—During fasting the body draws upon its own reserve of stored material for the requirements in the production of energy, and the rate of break-down varies with the energy requirements. An individual who is kept warm in bed, therefore, stands fasting longer than one who is compelled to take exercise in a cold place."

In Nelson's Encyclopœdia, Vol IV, p. 582, we read:

"The observations made during the fasts of Succi and others show that the body wastes less rapidly when the patient is kept warm and at rest."

It is very clear that nothing but a reduction of the number of calories of heat radiated, and hence consumed from reserve tissue to keep up body heat could account for "warmth" reducing the body waste as noted above. This is even more clearly shown in experiments of M. Chosset (Recherches experimentals sur l' inanition) quoted in the American Ency., Vol. I, p. 40, where it says that he "deprived a number of animals (birds and small mammals) of all sustenance and carefully observed the phenomena that followed, and his experiments throw much light upon the subject of starvation. The temperature in all the animals was maintained at nearly the normal standard until the last day of life, when it began rapidly to fall. The animals, previously restless now became quiet, as if stupefied; they fell over on their side unable to stand, the breathing became slower and slower, the pupils dilated, the insensibility grew more profound, and death took place either quietly or attended with convulsions. If when these phenomena were *fully developed,* external warmth was applied, the animals revived; their muscular force returned, they moved or flew about the room, and took *greedily* the food that was presented to them. If now they were again left to themselves they speedily perished; but *if the external temperature was maintained until the food taken was digested* (and from the feeble condition of their digestive organs this often took many hours) *they recovered. The immediate cause of death seemed to be cold rather than starvation.*"

The italics are the present writer's and show that warmth has a tremendous effect in prolonging life, even almost up to the last moment of life.

The present writer considers these statements conclusive evidence that some, at least, if not the larger part, of our food is used solely to keep up body warmth, consequently the only way the real minimum diet, such as would be required in the hottest summer weather, can be determined is by measuring the amount of tissue consumed by a person fasting, while inactive and kept at a temperature of 98.6° F. or higher, by artificial or summer heat. This would give approximately the minimum diet possible, to which later experiments might add the amount required for work and body warmth at different air temperatures.

A few crude experiments during hot weather led the present writer to believe that from 300 to 350 calories a day is about the minimum amount of food required to maintain the body structure of a 160-pound man, without making any allowance for the energy radiated as heat or used or expended as work by the body. Of course, everyone would have to eat enough to replace all tissue destroyed in working, but this varies so widely in different people, and from day to day, that probably the best indication of what should be eaten would be natural hunger and, of course, a continuously odorless excreta.

However, the writer has not been able to find any record of a diet so low; in fact, in Bulletins Nos. 77, 126 and 203 of the Carnegie Institute of Washington, a cursory examination has failed to show that any attention was paid to finding whether or not there was any relation between the differences in temperature between the air and the body, and the rate at which the body radiated or "lost" heat, although the statement is made in Bul. 126, p. 118, that

"The marvelous thing about it is that the two processes (the development of heat and the dissipation of heat) are ordinarily so delicately balanced."

In an article by Dr. J. Arthur Harris, and Dr. F. G. Benedict, p. 385 in the Scientific Monthly for May, 1919, the statement is made (p. 387) that

Physiologists have gradually come to a general agreement that the heat production at complete muscular repose and in the post-absorption state, i. e., about 12 hours after the last meal shall be called the basal metabolism and shall be used as a standard of comparison in the investigation of all the special problems of human nutrition. . . ."

This appears to take no notice of the temperature of the air at the time the heat production is measured, at all, nor is the temperature at which the experiments were made even stated, nor is there any statement that they were all made at any one temperature or reduced by calculation to a "basal" temperature. Why this omission?

In the writer's opinion this is a fundamental error that renders the experiments of no value at all in finding the proper amount of food for the body.

However, that the rate of loss of body heat as a measure of the heat production has had considerable study in the past is indicated by the statement, p. 395:

"Throughout the entire history of the investigation of the metabolism of the warm-blooded animals, the question of the relationship between the body surface area of the organism and its heat production has been a center of interest. Even before the development of adequate experimental methods of investigating the energy transformation which takes place in the body of the vertebrate organism, the possible relationship of body surface area to heat production was a subject of speculation. . . ."

"Newton's law of cooling made a strong appeal to the imagination of earlier physiological writers. It is not surprising that, impressed as they were by the relative constancy of body temperature in the warm-blooded animals, they conceived of heat production as proportional to heat loss as a means of maintaining constant body temperature, and came to look upon heat loss as determined by body surface area and to consider heat loss as determining in its turn heat production. . . ."

"It must be admitted that the 'body surface law' has given excellent results. If, however, there be no purely physiological basis for assuming a casual relation between body surface and heat production it would seem desirable, if possible, to replace this formula by a more rational one."

Where could anything be found *more rational* than this idea of the "earlier physiologists?" Why not determine once for all the effects of Newton's Law of Cooling? It will only require a few weeks' work to settle the question.

In this article they have measured the metabolism of about 239 men and women and 94 "infants" in which they found the *"average basal metabolism per 24 hours* is as follows:

For 136 men, 1631.74 calories.
For 103 women, 1349.19 calories.
For 51 male infants, 144.55 calories.
For 43 female infants, 140.37 calories.

They have analyzed these on the basis of the effects of body weight, stature and age, and area of body surface on the metabolism, and although these later might have been corrected to a uniform temperature of air, the present writer failed to find any note to this effect, consequently believes them to be grievously in error as an indication of the true "basal" metabolism.

They have apparently made no effort to ascertain what influence the fluctuations of temperature of the air might have on the loss of heat of the body, in spite of the suggestions of the prior physiologists referred to.

The Ency. Brit., Vol. XIII, p. 149, says under "Heat Transference":

"Newton's Law of Cooling.—There is one essential condition common to all three modes of heat-transference, namely, that they depend on difference of temperature, that the direction of the transfer of heat is always from hot to cold, and that the rate of transference is, for small differences, directly proportioned to the difference of temperature. Without difference of temperature there is no transfer of heat. When two bodies have been brought to the same temperature by conduction they are also in equilibrium as regards radiation, and vice versa . . . . the rate of cooling at any moment will be proportional to the difference of temperature. This simple relation is commonly known as 'Newton's Law of Cooling,' but is limited in its application to comparatively simple cases such as the foregoing."

In Carnegie Institute of Washington Pub. 77, Table 231, pp. 476-7 is published a resume of the heat lost by the body in different ways, in about 18 experiments; 14 made without food and 4 with food, none of which however were made in hot weather, but as these all show that practically ¾ of the heat eliminated was by radiation and conduction, the writer has compiled the following table of averages from this article.

TABLE OF THE AVERAGES OF HEAT ELIMINATED BY THE BODY IN DIFFERENT WAYS, AMOUNTS PER DAY AND PROPORTIONS OF TOTAL METABOLISM IN METABOLISM WITH AND WITHOUT FOOD—TAKEN FROM TABLE 231, PAGES 476-7, CARNEGIE INST. BUL. 77.

	Quantities of heat per day in calories							Proportion of total for 24 hours.					
	By radiation and conduction	Required to warm inspired air	In urine and feces	In water vaporised from lungs and skin			Total for 24 hours	By radiation and conduction	Required to warm inspired air	For urine and feces	In water vaporised from lungs and skin		
				From lungs	From skin	Total		%	%	%	From lungs %	From skin %	Total %
Average of 14 experiments without food (total 43 days)......	1440	44	22	185	239	424	1931	74.6	2.3	1.1	9.6	12.4	22.0
Averrge of 4 experiments with food (total 10 days)......	1374	43	23	185	227	408	1848	74.7	2.3	1.2	9.8	12.3	22.1

By "Newton's Law of Cooling" the loss of heat by radiation and conduction will be an entirely unnecessary expenditure of energy during the hot months of summer, at least in some parts of the country, and at times when the thermometer is above 99 degrees and, in fact, this item should vary throughout the year in close relation to the difference of temperature between the body and the surrounding air.

However, the present writer can find no evidence of this having been considered by Dr. Benedict, in these recent publications, and believes an experiment should be made, measuring a person's metabolism, with the body at rest, and kept at 99° F. by artificial heat, to prove or disprove his contention.

Should the writer's contention in this matter be correct, his estimate of 300 to 350 calories as being the "basal" metabolism for extremely hot weather should be approximately correct. This would account for the fact noted by the several authorities quoted that the application of external heat would much prolong life during a fast, and also explain why a young girl (Case No. 24) could live six months without food in Brazil, near the equator, without great loss in weight, while others might starve to death in 40 to 90 days in a colder climate. It would also indicate why an Eskimo can eat such quantities of meat and still never get cancer, as is claimed by opponents of the theory that excessive meat eating is the principal cause of cancer, the radiation of heat, of course, being very greatly increased by the extreme cold and hence utilizing the extra food in this manner.

Another thing which the present writer believes to be grievously in error is the idea of taking the *average* of the metabolism of these experiments as the "basal" metabolism. He believes the minimum is a far better guide as to what should be eaten and that the excreta should also be odorless as described by Horace Fletcher.

In these experiments described on page 112, 67 men or more unquestionably had a smaller metabolic rate than the average given of 1631.74 calories a day; one man having less than 1,012 calories a day, and a second man less than 1,087 calories a day, while the maximum was over 2,513 calories a day, or practically 2½ times as much. ·

The writer has seen a table posted in a railway roundhouse showing the amount of coal and oil used by each fireman on a locomotive during a month's time, which had a very similar range, the maximum used, if he remembers correctly, being well above twice the minimum, figured on a ton mile basis.

In this case no one would think of the tail end of the list (high consumption) nor even the average as representing first-class efficient work, and the writer believes the cases of high consumption in food are no more worthy of attention as efficient or correct diet, especially when a foul odor of the excreta is present, indicating that some of the food at least is wasted.

While the writer may be in error as to living on 300 or 350 calories of food during hot weather, he believes this is approximately correct considering the crudity of his experiments and also believes that a person should never eat except when urged by natural hunger or a feeling vastly different from the gluttonous hunger or craving which the ordinary person calls hunger. There is no weakness, no gnawing craving, no "all gone" feeling accompanying natural hunger. A person experiencing natural hunger feels a great buoyancy of spirit and strength and keenness of eyesight that, in the writer's opinion, can be obtained under no other conditions whatever.

By keeping in such condition that natural hunger will indicate when one should eat and not eating more than is required to just satisfy natural hunger, a person can live probably indefinitely, with perfectly odorless excreta and in the most abounding good health, entirely immune to all germ diseases.

However, if one overeats for a while, as is very likely during the cold months of the year, when much more food must be eaten than during summer, he should take a fast of sufficient length to bring natural hunger and odorless excreta again, when the weather warms up in the spring.

The writer, as will be noted, has placed all the emphasis on the quantity of food to be eaten, leaving a person to follow the indication of their natural hunger as to what to eat, and will only add on this subject that it is far better to confine oneself to foods that can be obtained in a natural condition, omitting entirely from the diet such foods as white flour bread, pastry, etc., in fact any food that has been denatured or robbed of its natural mineral salts.

He believes the hot weather diet should comprise about 300-350 calories, at least two-thirds of which should be protein food, the balance divided between fats and mineral salts, with practically no carbohydrates whatever, while, as cold weather comes on, a person should add to the above diet sufficient carbohydrates to keep up the body heat, and when called upon for extreme hard work an extra amount of food will also be required.

Prof. Chittenden concludes in "The Nutrition of Man" (pg. 274), that 60 gms. (2 oz.) of protein, when combined with the usual amounts of other kinds of food, is sufficient for bodily maintenance in a man weighting 70 kg. (154 lbs.) ; and the consumption of protein tissue by A. Levanzin during his fast, heretofore mentioned, was only slightly higher, and that of mineral salts only about ⅛ oz. daily.

During this fast, the consumption of carbohydrates was practically nothing, proving that the body can exist for some time without same, while the heat produced from fat was only a little below the amount of heat radiated, and this fat might have been burned principally to support body temperature, although *some* fat is necessary to support metabolism.

A very good discussion of individual foods and their uses and effects on the body will be found in "How to Stay Young," by Dr . Robt. B. Armitage, M. D.

For some time after fasting to natural hunger a person will have great difficulty in finding a diet upon which they can keep in good health, with odorless excreta and natural hunger, but the present writer is satisfied that it can be done, although he has not by any means entirely solved the diet problem yet.

However, by eating foods suuch as fruit, nuts, grains, vegetables, etc., in their natural states as nearly as possible, to preserve all the mineral salts they contain for the use of the body, a person should be able to attain very good health without following any "set" diet.

One or at most two meals a day should be enough.

CHAPTER X.

COMPULSORY VACCINATION IS UNCONSTITUTIONAL!
COMPULSORY HOSPITALIZATION IS ALSO UNCONSTITU-
TIONAL!

Stand upon your *Inalienable Rights* and refuse both.

The writer did not intend to start a legal treatise on
the rights of "Health" officers to coerce others, but in view
of our recent "orders" "requiring" the vaccination of
thousands of people, he believes something should be said
on the subject. "Compulsory" vaccination and hospitalization are subjects on which there is not a great amount of
knowledge among the lay people. The ordinary man, when
a "Health" officer comes blustering around, asserting he
has "police power" to do anything for the "common good,"
will allow him, often, to carry off his most cherished child
to the pesthouse or isolation hospital, to "forbid" the par-
ents seeing the child except as ordered by the "doctor," and
to force on the child any medicine, serum or vaccine that
the superstitious cowpox quack in charge may wish to
"try," to see if it won't cure some disease the victim may be
accused of having by the cowpox quacks of the "Health"
department; without knowing that no health officer has any
right to touch the body of himself or any member of his
family, or forcibly medicate, inoculate or vaccinate any one
against his will, under any conditions whatever.

The most complete discussion of a man's rights to
medical freedom, which the writer has seen is in the "Hor-
rors of Vaccination," by Mr. Charles M. Higgins, from
which most of the material quoted herein is taken, with
some rearrangement. Mr. Higgins bases his argument on
the following quotation from the Declaration of Independ-
ence, the substance of which is embodied in all state constitutions:

"We hold these truths to be self-evident, that all men
are created equal, that they are endowed by their Creator
with certain inalienable Rights, that among these are Life,

Liberty and the pursuit of Happiness. That to secure these rights, Governments are instituted among Men, deriving their just powers *from the consent of the governed. That whenever any Form of Government becomes destructive of these ends it is the* right of the People to alter or to abolish it." (Italics are ours.)

Mr. Higgins shows that Compulsory Vaccination, or other medical coercion of any kind, is a violation of a man's sovereign rights to his own body, rights "endowed by his Creator" and which our ancestors declared to be *"inalienable"* by any Government before they wrote the Constitution!

As Mr. Higgins also shows, after making this assertion that a man has certain *inherent and inalienable rights of which inviolability of person is one,* and after asserting *that government is instituted to secure these rights* of the individual and not to suppress them, our forefathers wrote into the Constitution, to further protect the people, the following:

Articles IX and X

IX. "The enumeration in the Constitution of certain rights, shall not be construed to deny or disparage others *retained by the people.*"

X. "The powers not delegated to the United States by the Constitution, nor prohibited by it to the States, are *reserved* to the States respectively, or *to the people.*"

As Mr. Higgins says:

"Here we plainly see that the Constitution, as well as the Declaration which preceded it, show that the People have a whole series of "certain," "inalienable," "reserved" and "retained" rights, and that these several rights, both specified and unspecified, *are divinely conferred and naturally inherent and cannot be invaded or taken away by any government, but must be respected, defended and enforced by all governments, and that governments exist for the chief purpose of defending and enforcing these rights.*"

Daniel Webster, the famous American Statesman, once said:

"Compulsory vaccination is an outrage and a gross interference with the liberty of the people in a land of freedom."

Prof. F. W. Newman of Oxford University (Eng.) has said:

"Against the body of a healthy man Parliament has no right of assault whatever under pretense of the Public Health; nor any the more against the body of a healthy infant. To forbid perfect health is a tyrannical wickedness, just as much as to forbid chastity or sobriety. No lawgiver can have the right. The law is an unendurable usurpation. and creates the right of resistance."

On this point, Blackstone. the English law commentator, says:

"No laws are binding on the human subject which assault the body or violate the conscience."

Court Decisions Upon the Subject

Now that we have seen upon what grounds a man can refuse vaccination against his will, let us see what some of the courts say on the question. Massachusetts passed a statute requiring the vaccination of all persons in good health, under penalty of a fine of $5.00 for refusing vaccination.

.The Supreme Court of the State, in the case of Jacobson in 1904, said:

"If a person deem it important that vaccination should not be performed in his case and the authorities should think otherwise, *it is not in their power to vaccinate him by force,* and the worst that could happen to him under the statute would be the payment of the penalty of five dollars." (183 Mass. 242.)

Upon appeal of this case the United States Supreme Court said in 1905 in affirming the decision:

"There is, of course, a sphere within which the individual may assert the supremacy of his own will and rightfully dispute the authority of any human government, especially of any free government existing under a written constitution, to interfere with the exercise of that will," (197 U. S. 11)

and further held, apparently, that, *if he had proved that vaccination was dangerous to health and life, he could not even have been fined for refusing it,* although it approved the lower court's ruling out apparently as improper, all evidence as to the effects of vaccination that was offered.

But this decision in spite of these views, supported the constitutionality of the Massachusetts Statute, principally on the ground that it is a matter of "common belief" that vaccination prevents smallpox and is not injurious; for instance, in approving the lower court's rejection of the defendant's "proofs" to the contrary, the judge said:

"Those offers in the main seem to have had no purpose except to state the general theory of those of the medical profession who attach little or no value to vaccination as a means of preventing the spread of smallpox, or who think that vaccination causes other diseases of the body." "What everybody knows the court must know, and therefore the state court judicially, as this court knows, that an opposite *theory* accords with the common belief, and is maintained by high medical authority. We must assume that when the statute in question was passed the legislature of Massachusetts was not unaware of these opposing theories, and was compelled of necessity, to choose between them. It was not compelled to commit a matter involving the public health and safety to the final decision of a court. It is no part of the function of a court or jury to determine which one of two modes was likely to be the most effective for the protection of the public against disease. That was for the legislative department to determine in the light of all the information it had or could obtain." . . .

"Whatever may be thought of the expediency of this statute it cannot be affirmed to be beyond question, in palpable conflict with the Constitution." "Nor in view of the methods employed to stamp out the disease of smallpox, can anyone confidently assert that the means prescribed by the state to that end has no real or substantial relation to the protection of the public health and the public safety." (197 U. S. 11.)

And they admit themselves that this view is founded upon a *theory,* supported by *common belief,* and the statements of the *serum sellers and vaccine venders themselves,* and assume to rule out of the evidence all the proofs to the contrary offered by the defendant. It may be that these proofs were improperly presented and hence inadmissible but, is there any more justice in such a decision, than there

would be in letting patent medicine manufacturers or sales-
men, in a similar suit, place their testimonials on the records and reject all testimony opposing their views? And
this decision comes many years after Dr. Charles Creighton, the famous English physician, said:

*"The anti-vaccinationists have knocked the bottom out
of a GROTESQUE SUPERSTITION."* ("Jenner and Vaccination." 1879.)

Regarding Jacobson's proofs of the injurious or dangerous effects the Court said in effect:

"Each of them, in its nature, is such that it cannot be
stated as a truth, otherwise than as a matter of opinion.
The only 'competent evidence' that could be presented to the
Court to prove these propositions was the testimony of experts, giving their opinions. It would not have been competent to introduce the medical history of individual cases.
Assuming that medical experts could have been found who
would have testified in support of these propositions, and it
had become the duty of the Judge . . .   to instruct the
jury as to whether or not the statute is constitutional, he
would have been obliged to consider the evidence in connection with facts of common knowledge, which the court will
always regard in passing upon the constitutionality of a
statute. He would have considered this testimony of experts in connection with the facts that for nearly a century
most of the members of the medical profession have regarded
vaccination, repeated at intervals, as a preventive of smallpox; that while they have recognized the possibility of
injury . . .   they generally have considered the risk
 . . .   too small to be seriously weighed against the benefits coming from the discreet and proper use of the preventive;
and that not only the medical profession and the people
generally have for a long time entertained these opinions,
but legislatures and courts have acted upon them with general
unanimity." (197 U. S. 11.)

Would not this opinion make *witchcraft* perfectly lawful and constitutional, provided it was a matter of "common opinion" that it was a cure? Why do not our courts
take the stand that if there is a difference of opinion, and
if vaccination really does protect, those vaccinated would
be protected by *their own* vaccination, and hence any one

who knows how useless and dangerous it really is, *should be protected in their desire to be let alone.*

In another case, that of the Union Pacific Railway vs. Botsford, the United States Supreme Court says:

" . . . No right is held more sacred or is more carefully guarded by the common law, than the right of every individual to the possession and control of his own person, free from all restraint or interference of others unless by clear and unquestionable authority of law." As well said by Judge Cooley: "The right of one's person may be said to be a right of complete immunity; to be let alone." (Cooley on Torts, 29.)

"The inviolability of the person is as much invaded by a compulsory stripping as by a blow. To compel any one, and especially a woman, to lay bare the body or to submit it to the touch of a stranger, without lawful authority, is an indignity, an assault, and a trespass." (141 U. S. 250.)

In another case, Judge Gaynor, of the New York Supreme Court, in the case of Smith against Health Commissioner Emery, of Brooklyn, in 1894, gave the following decision which was afterwards fully sustained by the New York Court of Appeals:

"If the Commissioner (of Health) had the power to imprison an individual for refusing to submit to vaccination, I see no reason why he should not also imprison one for refusing to swallow a dose. But the Legislature has conferred no such power upon him, *if, indeed, it has the power to do the like.*" . . . "If the legislature desired to make vaccination compulsory it would have so enacted. Whether it be within its power to do so, and if so, by what means it may enforce such an enactment, are not for discussion here." (84 Hun. 570.)

Two years later in 1896 (before Judge Brown) Mr. Smith recovered $489.00 damages against Health Commissioner Emery for false imprisonment and illegal quarantine, while in 1895 (in the Supreme Court of Brooklyn) another party named Schaeffer recovered $1,500.00 damages against Commissioner Emery's assistant for forcible vaccination of himself and family.

This decision asserts clearly a man's right to refuse

any medical treatment he does not wish to take, regardless
of the doctor's opinion that it is necessary, consequently he
would have the same right to refuse forcible "hospitalization."

Again, 9 years later, Judge Woodward of the New
York Appellate Court, in the Viemeister case in 1903, declared that:

"It may be conceded that the Legislature has no constitutional right to compel any person to submit to vaccination." (84 N. Y. Supp. 712.)

At the second trial of the Bollinger case, in the Supreme Court, Columbia County, N. Y., in 1910, Judge
Le Boeuf charged the jury, partly, as follows:

"Now, I have charged you that this assault which is
claimed to have existed here, due to the forcible vaccination, that is, if it was against this man's will, is one which
you must consider. And the reason of that is: *This man,
in the eyes of the law, just as you and I and all of us in this
court-room, has the right to be let alone. We all have the
right to the freedom of our persons and that freedom of our
persons may not be unlawfully invaded. That is a great
right. It is one of the most important rights we have.*"
(Italics are ours.)

This is a very clear statement of our inalienable rights
—the right all of us have to be let alone.

And this right of course is inherent in every American
citizen whether in school, in the U. S. Army, Navy or Ma-
rines, or employed where the "Health" officers may "order"
or "advise" vaccination.

Neither have any so-called "Health" officers the right
to forcibly "hospitalize" or shanghai any one to enforce
the use of their drugs, serums or vaccines, against the patient's wishes, and any use of coercion by "Health" officers,
or employers, etc., renders them liable for damages.

A man has the right to use as much force as may be
necessary to prevent any so-called "Health" officer's seiz-
ing or attempting to seize his person or the persons of his
children, and in fact such attempts persisted in would jus-

tify any action taken in self defense, and no show of badges, assertion of "police power," or the presence of uniformed policemen, affects that right in any way whatever.

In fact our policemen should be informed as to a person's inalienable rights, and instructed to prevent such acts, instead of lending assistance by their presence.

In Illinois we have no State Laws "compelling" vaccination, but there are some local ordinances assuming to do this and regarding these we have one important decision at least.

Judge Cartwright, of the Illinois Supreme Court, in the case of The People ex rel, Louise Jenkins, Appellant, vs. The Board of Education et al, Appellees, a case resulting from expulsion from school for refusal to be vaccinated, handed down an important decision, April 23, 1908, of which the following are a few excerpts:

"Not only has the legislature never prescribed vaccination as a condition to the enjoyment of the legal right to attend public schools, but they have never conferred upon cities the power to do so."

Of a section of a Chicago City Ordinance, which said:

"No principal or person in charge or control of any school shall admit to such school any child who shall not have been vaccinated within seven years preceding the admission or application for admission to any such school of such child, nor shall any such principal or person retain in or permit to attend any such school any child who shall not have been vaccinated as provided in this article." (Sec. 1255.)

He declared

"section 1255 (above) is null and void and affords no justification for denying relator admission to school. Whether the denial of her legal right was at the instance of the health commissioner, the health department or any other authority."

He also said:

"The general police powers above enumerated to pass ordinances and make regulations for the promotion of health or the suppression of disease do not include the passage of such an ordinance as this, which makes vaccination a condition precedent to the right to an education." . . .

"The health commissioner is a purely ministerial officer and has no legislative powers whatever. The ordinance Sec. 1035, does not purport to give him authority to exercise such powers or to make any rules or regulations except in cases of emergency, until they can be reported to the city council for approval or rejection.

"There is nothing in the nature of an emergency in the occasional recurrence of the well known disease of smallpox in a city like Chicago which may not be provided for by general rules and regulations prescribed by the legislative authority of the city, (instead of attempting to delegate to the health commission the power to make emergency rules when the disease appears.)

"The Board of Education, which has charge of the public schools, has made no rule or regulation on the subject of such epidemics, and neither has the city council. The answer does not make known any ordinance, rule or regulation for the exclusion from the schools of children not vaccinated in the event that an epidemic of smallpox exists in the vicinity of a school or is reasonably apprehended, and in our opinion the (lower)court erred in overruling the demurrer." (234 Ill. 422.)

(Demurrer was to the "setting up in justification of the exclusion of the relator" an ordinance of the city of Chicago and instructions by the health department to enforce such ordinance.)

However, there is a later decision which *seems* contrary to this idea of the matter, namely, that of Clifton Hagler et al, Appellants, vs. R. H. Larner, et al, Appellees, appealed from the City Court of Granite City.

This seems completely to support the health boards' right to "order" "compulsory" vaccination as a condition of school attendance, although in reality it does not do this. The plaintiffs contended the health board's order was a legislative action, and therefore unconstitutional and the court decided that being a temporary order only, it was an administrative action and therefore within the boards' constitutional powers. The decision is also based upon the absolutely false assumption that vaccination "prevents" smallpox, and with this proven false, it would have no grounds to stand on. Furthermore, it is only under conditions similar to those prevalent in Granite City, at the time the order was issued, namely, 40 cases of smallpox in 12,000 population, that it held the order to be reasonable. Hence it is not comparable with conditions where there is no such epidemic.

The decision said in part:

"The resolution of the board of health was reasonable in view of the fact that smallpox was epidemic and the disease likely to spread from the many cases then existing in the city. *It is not disputed that the purpose of the board of health in passing the resolution was the prevention of the spread of the disease and preserving the health of the citizens, and there is no argument offered by appellants that that would not be its tendency or that the actual express purpose of the board would not be accomplished by the enforcement of the board's rule.* The requirement of the resolution was that such exclusion of the pupils should be temporary or for two weeks, and then only in case they refused to be vaccinated, etc. The only objection to the resolution, in fact, is that the board had no sufficient authority to pass the same and the school board was therefore without power to enforce it. . . . The rule adopted by the board was not a permanent rule or law, but a mere temporary order set in force for a limited time as a means of stamping out smallpox and preventing the further spread thereof in said city. The rule or regulation expired at the expiration of the limit fixed for it to remain in force and cannot in any sense be said to be a legislative act. *No one was compelled to be vaccinated.* The simple effect of the order was that no child could enter the school unless vaccinated while the rule of the board requiring vaccination was in force. . . . No child has a constitutional right to carry to others in school the loathsome disease of smallpox. Vaccination is now recognized as the only safe prevention of the spread of smallpox. It is approved by medical science generally and by governmental authorities throughout the civilized world. In many countries compulsory vaccination has become the settled policy of the State, and our own country has adopted it as one of the preliminary requisites to military service. . . . By the teachings of the best medical authorities a person who has been thoroughly and successfully vaccinated will be entirely immune from the disease or put in such condition that if the should contract the disease it would only be in the very mild form, commonly known as varioloid, which rarely occasions scarring or fatal results. In other words the result of vaccination, according to such authorities, is not only the arrest of the spreading of the disease, but the prevention of fatalities among those who are actually exposed to the disease and who contract it in its milder form. While on the other hand, it is true that occasionally very disastrous results happen from the use of impure vaccine, and there are many people for that or other reasons, who resist, and *have the right to resist*, compulsory vaccination of their children except in cases of 'necessity, yet they have no right to insist on their children continuing in school and mixing in large congregations without obeying such requirements when smallpox is epidemic in the community and such children perhaps been exposed to the same." (284 Ill. 547.) (Italics are ours.)

They do not seem to realize that if *those who wanted protection were vaccinated*, they should be immune to the exposure caused by associating with unvaccinated people, if vaccination was of any use.

Most other decisions supporting compulsory vaccination also appear to be based upon this false assumption that vaccination "prevents" smallpox without causing any other harm, and of course must be reversed when the "common belief" on this point is reversed, which the writer hopes will be very soon.

A clever man has said:

"When a dentist makes a mistake, the patient loses his tooth; when a doctor makes a mistake, he buries it; when a judge makes a mistake, it becomes the law."

Does it not seem extremely far fetched and indicate prejudice on the part of the court to base such important decisions, concerning a man's constitutional rights, on "common belief," in the face of overwhelming evidence that such common belief is no more than a "Grotesque Superstition"; and even to rule out evidence that would prove vaccination injurious and useless on the ground that (as the U. S. Supreme Court said in the Jacobson case):

"These offers seem to have had no purpose, except to state the general theory of those—who attach little or no value to vaccination."

The Supreme Court of Florida, however, seems to take a somewhat different view as to a man's constitutional rights to choose any method of treatment he wishes: in a recent decision, that of Bradley vs. State, a case in which a man was prosecuted because his child had died of burns, after being three weeks without medical attention; it said in part:

"The all-important question is: must a parent call a physician every time his child is sick, or risk being adjudged guilty of manslaughter if the child should die? If not, who is to decide when the child is sick enough to place upon the father the obligation to call a physician? Is it the father, or the neighbors, or must the father call a physician to ascertain if the child needs a physician?

"Has the practice of medicine become an exact science, so that after death, human testimony can establish beyond a reasonable doubt that if a physician had been called the child would not have died?

"Does the duty of the parent to call a physician attach where a child is afflicted with a necessarily fatal ailment, such as consumption, and continue until death occurs? Can the law fix what class of ailments a child must be suffering from before the failure to call a physician becomes culpable negligence, so that if death ensues in one class it is manslaughter and in another class it is not? Shall a parent, who belongs to that exemplary band of Christians who have no faith in the efficacy of medicine as a curative agency, be convicted of manslaughter because he fails to call a physician to attend a sick child that subsequently dies? Until the practice of medicine becomes an exact science so that it can be established beyond the peradventure of a doubt that death would not have ensued if a physician had been in attendance, I think the answer to all these questions must be an unqualified 'NO.' "

"The reasoning upon which the State's case rests is this: The child was badly injured; it did not have medical attention for three weeks; after that it was in the care of a physician for two weeks before it died; if the father had called a physician it would have recovered; therefore the refusal of the father to call a physician caused the child's death. The fallacy of this is that it was not proven, and was not capable of being proven, that if the child had had medical attention it would have recovered. And that must always be the fallacy in an attempt to attach the guilt of manslaughter to a father for failing to call a physician whenever his child is sick if it subsequently dies." (84 So. 677.)

Would that we had more courts that would take similar views!

The allopathic doctors, however, are doing everything possible to get laws passed both in Congress and in the various State Legislatures that will give them absolute power over all "health" measures and all treatment of disease, and are using every means to spread their serum propaganda wherever possible.

There is a bill (S. B. 363) now pending before the Illinois State Senate that makes it murder or manslaughter to allow a child to die without a so-called "regular" doctor in attendance; a bill which would deprive 100% of our population of the right to have any treatment for disease except the serums, antitoxins and drugs of the allopathic school of medicine and they are trying to get their members in all public offices where they can increase the sale of their devilish serums, etc.

It is time for the public to call a halt; fight the allopaths to a finish; repeal the license laws that give them their hold, and pass laws to bar all graduates from medical schools from holding a position as "Health" officer any place in the U. S. A.

Suits for damages should also be filed against all employers who discharge, or refuse to employ anyone, because they refuse vaccination. This would soon put a damper on this practice.

Not until then will our constitutional rights to choose our methods of treating disease be safe.

On June 22, 1921, the Illinois Medical Practice Act as revised in 1917, was found unconstitutional in the State Supreme Court in the case of Dr. L. J. Love, a chiropractor of Danville, who was refused the right to be examined as a Chiropractor because he had no medical training. The opinion of the court, written by Justice Duncan, and concurred in by the full membership of the bench, held that the revisions of requirements for chiropractic are unreasonable and discriminatory.

The old law (now restored by the decision) did not specify what qualifications were required to obtain a license as chiropractor, and the revised law required a course of study equivalent to that of the so-called "regular" physicians in addition to their chiropractic training.

APPENDIX A.

More Information on the Germ Theory and Vaccination.

Since paging up Chapter III the writer has found additional information to support the idea that vaccination only modifies the "characteristics" of the germ, thus changing, what would otherwise appear to be one disease, into another having more or less different "characteristics" thus accounting for such diseases as "sleeping sickness" and other more or less "mysterious" diseases so-called.

Allow us to remind you again that the Ency. Brit., Vol. 3, p. 172d, under Bacteriology, says:

"As our knowledge has advanced it has become abundantly evident that the so-called pathogenic bacteria are not organisms with special features, but that each is a member of a group of organisms possessing closely allied characters. From the point of view of evolution we may suppose that certain races of a group of bacteria have gradually acquired the power of invading the tissues of the body and producing disease. In the acquisition of pathogenic properties some of their original characters have become changed, *but in many instances this has taken place only to a light degree, and furthermore, some of these changes are not of a permanent character.* It is to be noted that in the case of bacteria we can only judge of organisms being of different species by the stability of the characters which distinguish them and *numerous examples might be given where their characters become modified by comparatively slight change in their environment. The cultural as well as the microscopical characters of a pathogenic organism may be closely similar to other non-pathogenic members of the same group, and it thus becomes a matter of extreme difficulty in certain cases . . . . in differentiating varieties.*"

In "Facts and Comments," published in 1902, Mr. Herbert Spencer, the famous philosopher, discusses vaccination as follows:

"Jenner and his disciples have assumed that when the

vaccine virus has passed through a patient's system he is safe against smallpox, and there the matter ends. . . . . I merely propose to show that there the matter does *not* end. The interference with the order of Nature has various sequences other than that counted upon.

"A Parliamentary Return issued in 1880 (No. 392) shows that comparing the quinquennial periods of 1847-51 and 1874-8 there was in the latter a diminution in the deaths from all causes of infants under one year old of 6,600 per million births per annum; while the mortality caused by eight specified diseases either directly communicable or exacerbated by the effects of vaccination increased from 20,524 to 41,353 per million births per annum—more than double. It is clear that far more were killed by these other diseases than were saved from smallpox. . . . . . You cannot change the constitution in relation to one invading agent and leave it unchanged, in regard to all other invading agents. . . . . .

"There are, however, evidences of a general relative debility. Measles is a severer disease than it used to be, and deaths from it are very numerous. Influenza yields proof. Sixty years ago, when at long intervals an epidemic occurred it seized but few, was not severe, and left no serious sequelae; now it is permanently established, affects multitudes in extreme forms, and often leaves damaged constitutions. The disease is the same but there is less ability to withstand it." . . . . .

He quotes friends to show that vaccination does not prevent smallpox, and ascribes much of the prevalent poor teeth, health and eyesight to the weakened condition resulting from vaccination, and says:

"Be these suggestions true or not one thing is certain: the assumption that vaccination changes the constitution in relation to smallpox and does not otherwise change it is sheer folly."

Spencer made these statements eighteen years ago, yet we still have with us an enormously powerful medical clique still doing their best to foist upon the long-suffering public their damnable vaccines.

Paratyphoids were never reported in the Reports of the Surgeon General of the U. S. Army until inoculation against typhoid was introduced in 1909; now they are a separate disease recognized and classified to the extent of 21 varieties, by at least one authority the writer has seen.

If vaccination against typhoid does not prevent any paratyphoid and vaccination against typhoid and one paratyphoid does not prevent another, would not at least 22 separate and distinct vaccines be required to prevent all of them, and thus make a man safe?

In U. S. Public Health Reports, Vol. 34 (March 28, 1919) p. 611, they say (quoting from a circular issued by the chief surgeon of the A. E. F.) :

"In view of the fact that the ordinary clinical picture of typhoid-paratyphoid is very frequently *profoundly modified in vaccinated individuals*, it is considered essential to enumerate briefly the usual clinical manifestations of these fevers, atypical modes of onset, differential diagnosis and modifications of the usual clinical manifestations in vaccinated individuals."

Isn't it very likely that when a person was vaccinated against all of these the microscopic picture would be so profoundly modified as to show some varieties not yet known?

The writer is satisfied that *all* paratyphoids are merely modified or transitory forms of typhoid caused by vaccination, and as fast as new vaccines are discovered and applied, new paratyphoids, or entirely new diseases, will also be "discovered," such as sleeping sickness.

The Journal of the American Medical Association says in the issue for Sept. 11, 1920, p. 755:

The Great Influenza Epidemic (In England)

A further report on the great influenza epidemic of 1918-1919, issued by the registrar-general, brings out several most interesting points. The deaths numbered 112,329, for males being 53,883 and for females 58,446. The males included 7,591 noncivilians, and, deducting these, the deaths of civilians corresponded to a mortality of 3,129 per million civilian population. No such mortality has ever before been recorded for any epidemic in this country since registration commenced, except in the case of the cholera epidemic of 1849, when the mortality from that cause rose to 3,033 per million population. None of the previous outbreaks of influenza can compare in mortality with that of 1918-1919. During the forty-six weeks from June 23 to May 10, the total deaths allocated to the disease were 151,446, including 140,989 of civilians, the corresponding civilian death rate for these forty-six weeks being at the annual rate of 4,774 per million population. The mortality attributed to influenza does not represent the whole of that caused by it. The entries under other headings, especially those of respiratory disease, were always bound to increase during an epidemic; and though that did not occur in 1918 to the same extent as in other recent outbreaks, allowance must be made for these increases in mortality, allocated to other causes, but really attributable to influenza, in endeavoring to measure the loss of life caused by the epidemic. An astonishing feature was the sudden change of age incidence. In earlier years, influenza was less important under 55 years and more so above that period. In 1918-1919, this position was suddenly reversed. *Those under 35 died in appalling numbers; those over 55 seemed to be relatively safe.* It may be doubted whether so sudden and so complete a change of incidence can be paralleled in the history of any other disease; yet all the weight of medical testimony goes to show that the influenza of 1918 was essentially the same as that of former years. Attempts have been made to explain the change as due to alteration in the circumstances of the population. Thus it has been suggested that aggregation of young women in munition works in 1918 may partly account for their specially heavy mortality. No simple explanation on these lines is possible. The alteration in age incidence accompanying the increased prevalence and fatality of the disease in 1918 seems to be more easily explained by a sudden change in the infecting organism than in the soil provided for its growth. We are thus left with the question, "What are the causes which from time to time endow a comparatively harmless malady with ferocious strength, enabling it to destroy its thousands of victims?" These causes may lie in the resisting power of the population; more probably they lie in the attacking power of the germ. If we could gain some idea of the principles at work it might be possible, in the future, to protect ourselves against another such calamity.

The report of the Ministry of "Health" contains the startling statement that "during the space of a few months the disease claimed a larger number of victims than fell during the whole of the European War."

Before the appalling visitation the medical profession practically confeses its powerlessness and perplexity. Yet the drugless doctors all show a death rate in influenza of 1 per cent or less. Read the writer's discussion of the transformation of typhoid and other diseases to influenza through modification of the germs characteristics in Chapter III, especially pages 37-8-9, and note the statement of Herbert Spencer above.

However this is not all. *The death rate from influenza at the Cook County Hospital for 1918 as given in their annual report was 39.2%*; that from Tuberculosis of the Lungs at this same hospital was given as 54% in the same report, and they are shanghaiing patients, sometimes at the point of a gun, to take that kind of treatment.

The writer believes these high death rates are primarily due to the neglect of proper sanitary measures toward the bowels, i. e., the failure to use frequent enemas.

Dr. Victor C. Vaughan says in Protein Split Products in relation to immunity and disease (p. 439) :

"In the inability of the bacterial cell to grow in the animal body either because it cannot feed upon the proteins of the body, or because it is itself destroyed by the ferments elaborated by the body cells lies the fundamental explanation of all forms of bacterial immunity either natural or acquired."

It seems to the writer that he is always perfectly immune to germ action when his excrement is perfectly odorless, but never so when it is not in this condition.

Dr. John Long, of London, Eng., in "Medical Priesthood," says he finds that frequent purging of the bowels greatly reduces the death rate in peritonitis, and the present writer believes the very frequent intestinal hemorrhages and perforations, which accompanied so many cases of typhoid and influenza in the A. E. F., were due almost entirely to the neglect of proper cleansing of the bowels by the allopathic doctors in charge.

The Truth Teller, of Battle Creek, in its issue of Feb. 22nd, '21, mentions the death of Gov. Parkhurst of Maine of "pneumonia" after receiving "massive doses of anti-toxin" for a "diphtheritic" infection under the tongue and says in part:

Rapid work for pneumonia you will say! Indeed far too rapid! A condition resembling pneumonia very closely, frequently follows anti-toxin administration. Many times it is fatal. We have the records of hundreds of such cases.

In "Vaccines and Serums Viewed From the Standpoint of Many Physicians," published by the Vivisection Investigation League, New York City, Dr. J. Edward Herman, M. D., is quoted as saying in a paper read before the Brooklyn Pathological Society and published in Medical Record, May 27, 1899: "Before anti-toxin was used in the Willard Parker Hospital, 16 per cent of the fatal cases died of pneumonia. During nine months of 1895, 53 per cent of the deaths were caused by this disease. Winters thought

'the enormous increase of pneumonia has no other explanation than the hypodermic injection of serum.'"

This book should be read by every person who wants to know what the various serums, anti-toxins, salvarsans, etc., used by the allopaths really do in the system.

Dr. Henry E. Lahn, M. D., notes in his book "Diagnosis from the Eye" (now called "Iriodology") that vaccination increases diphtheria while preventing smallpox, in the following words:

(pp. 27 of 1st Ed.) "The body of the child tries to eliminate the poison (vaccine) as diphtheria. *It is a well known fact that only vaccinated children get diphtheria, and*

that the disease is spreading with vaccination against small-pox. To exchange diphtheria for smallpox is certainly not wise; for it is self-evident that it is easier for the system to eliminate morbid matter if the latter is distributed all over the body where it has a large surface for its elimination, as in the case of smallpox—than if a small and moreover so very delicate part as the larynx is used for that purpose."

This statement (made in 1904), as does that of Herbert Spencer quoted above, anticipates the present writer by many years in the idea that *Vaccines and Serums only modify the Germ's Characteristics,* thus making any illness, or its "clinical picture", appear to have "characteristics" different from those of the disease against which one is *"protected."*

Yet our modern so-called "Health" officers are daily making greater efforts to "compel" everyone to take these damnable poisons or be thrown out of work or out of school.

APPENDIX B.

Eye Diagnosis

Since the body of this book was written the writer has heard of a (to him) new method of diagnosis of disease through markings, or discolorations on the iris of the eye.

It appears that the normal color of the iris in all pure blooded descendants of the Keltic and Indo-Caucasian races, is Azure Blue, and a pure light brown for the yellow, black and Indian races, and mixtures, and any appearance of another color is a sign of disease of some kind in some part of the body: For instance Brown Eyes, in the pure blooded descendants of the Keltic or Indo-Caucasian races, are an indication of auto-intoxication, and when this is cured the iris will again turn blue.

In a similar way every disease produces certain recognizable discolorations in a part of the iris sensitive to the influences of the organ or part affected; these effects are similar in man and animal, and have been studied, mapped and described in thousands of cases, so that anyone acquainted with the relations between the disease and the markings in the eye can tell from these what the disease is, although it requires some study and experience in the matter to get accuracy.

A broken bone will cause a black radial mark in the part of the iris related to the part of the body affected and this will be overgrown with white as it heals. Any torn tissue, and any incoordination or irritation will show similar white lines on healing.

Apparently food and vegetable products that can be absorbed and utilized by the body, do not show in the iris (except when auto-intoxication occurs, as noted above), but most poisons taken into the body do leave an indelible trace on the iris of the eye.

The effects of poisons can even be distinguished by inexperienced persons because the poisons leave their mark

in more prominent colors. The effects of any one poison
are also strikingly uniform in different persons' eyes, even
though it is administered in medicinal doses by the allopaths, and the part of the iris affected indicates the part
of the body most affected by the poison.

The writer has taken this information and that which
follows from three very valuable books: "Iridology, by Dr.
H. E. Lahn (1st Ed. 1904), "The Diagnosis from the
Eye," by Nils Liljquist (1916), and "Iridiagnosis," by Dr.
Henry Lindlahr (1919), and an article written by Dr. H.
H. Lynn of Buffalo, N. Y., in the Truth Teller for March
7, 1921.

A very few of the more commonly used allopathic
"remedies" and their effects on the system and markings on
the iris are as follows:

Antikamnia, Antifebrin, Antipyrin, Phenacetin, and
other similar coal tar products used in *headache powders,*
etc., are all insanity producers and cause a sort of white
wash looking veil in the upper part of the iris when accumulated in the system.

Arsenic (used in *Salversan*) shows like snowflakes in
the iris when retained in the system. It is a deadly poison
that does more harm than good.

Bromides paralyze the brain and appear in the iris
as a white crescent in the upper part of the iris.

Iodine drys up and affects the glandular organs and
causes red and brownish red spots, mostly in the parts of
the iris that correspond to the stomach, kidneys and brain.
Often around the iodine spots are found the white clouds
of a latent inflammation.

Lead gives the region of the stomach in the iris a
lead gray color.

Mercury, one of the allopaths' commonest "curealls,"
used both internally and externally, produces during the
first few years whitish-grey clouds, or a greyish white
crescent in the upper part of the iris as it affects the brain
first, then the lungs, after five or six years' use of same
or when large quantities have accumulated, there appears
near the outer edge of the iris of the blue eye a greyish-

white ring of a metallic shine, which looks somewhat blue in the brown eye. Locomotor ataxia, softening of the brain, etc., will develop in the later stages and death will soon follow unless something is done to purge the system of the mercury.

It is eliminated from the body through carbuncles, wart-like fistules, and mucous patches in the mouth or nose or blackish coverings which slowly separate from the skin.

Quinine in small quantities gives the part of the iris corresponding to the bowels a distinct yellow color; but if the whole body is saturated with the poison the yellow in the iris becomes predominant, the blue eye takes a greenish color, while the brown eye becomes somewhat more fallow. This drug occasionally causes complete deafness and often headaches, ringing in the ears, dullness and an intense desire to waste and destroy.

Strychnine, a so-called "heart tonic", is so poisonous the heart *must* drive it off, and hence is stimulated like calomel stimulates the bowels, *to get rid of it at all costs.* This poison causes a small white wheel around the pupil, with distinct white spokes and rim.

Vaccination against smallpox causes a darkening of the color of the iris beginning around the pupil, indicating a general deterioration of the system, particularly the lymph and blood.

It seems astonishing to the present writer that such a simple and accurate method of diagnosis as this is should not be looked into and used by the so-called "regular" physicians, but such appears to be the case.

In the Journal of the American Medical Association for December 28th, 1912, Dr. R. C. Cabot of the Massachusetts General Hospital, states that in 3,000 post mortems held upon cases who died in the Massachusetts General Hospital, the ante-mortem diagnosis was wrong in about 47% of the cases, *or over* 1,400 *of* 3,000 *cases died after being treated for a different disease than the one which caused death.*

The error was very small in the more slowly developing diseases, that for typhoid being given as 6%, while more acute diseases had a very much higher rate of error, for instance the errors in some cases were:

Broncho-pneumonia, errors.......... 67%
Vertebral Tuberculosis, errors........77%
Chronic Myocarditis, errors.........78%
Hepatic Abscess and Acute Pericarditis, errors 80%
Acute Nephritis, errors.............84%

Dr. Cabot says in part:

"The table represents the success and failure of certain methods rather than of certain men"—

"They mirror the methods of an average up to date American hospital"—

"Again, diseases that kill so quickly that the period of observation is very brief and the history often faulty or lacking altogether, will always show a large percentage of diagnostic failure."

Yet Eye Diagnosis will almost always indicate the organs affected on first inspection, and will generally give an expert in the art a very good idea of the nature of the trouble, whether it is poison, or disease, etc.—whether a bone is broken, etc., and should save 90% of the errors—where the errors are greatest; in acute diseases, cracked skull, internal injuries, etc.

As it is 41 years since the first book on this subject was written, and there are now three very good books on the subject in English, (Dr. Lahn's, being 17 years old) the writer believes a law should be passed barring from practice, say in six months after passage, all physicians who cannot pass an examination in this subject.

BIBLIOGRAPHY ON FASTING.

Densmore, Emmet, M. D.
"*How Nature Cures.*"

Haskell, C. C., M. D., Norwich, Conn.
"*Perfect Health.*"

Keith, Geo. S., M. D., LL. D., F. R. C. P. E. (Scotland).
"*Plea for a Simple Life and Fads of An Old Physician.*"

Shew, D.
"*The Family Physician.*"

Gunn, R. A.
"Forty Days Without Food," by Robert A. Gunn, 1880, published by Albert Metz & Co., 60 John St., New York, describes a 42 days fast in Minneapolis in 1877 and a 40-day fast in New York in 1880 by Mr. H. S. Tanner, latter one watched continuously, the author being one of the watchers; 4¼ in. by 7¼ in.; 106 pp.

Dewey, E. H., M. D.
"The True Science of Living," 1894, by Dr. E. H. Dewey, M. D., Meadville, Pa.

A description of Dr. Dewey's discovery of the fasting treatment for the cure of disease and cases treated with supporting evidence that this is Nature's method. A series of lectures in printed form.

1894; 5½ x 8¾ inches; 323 pp.; Pub. C. C. Haskell & Son, Norwich, Conn.

Dewey, E. H., M. D.
"The No Breakfast Plan and the Fasting Cure," by E. H. Dewey, M. D., 1900, Meadville, Pa. A short description of Dr. Dewey's fasting and dieting plan, describing various cases, etc. A good book, although Dr. Dewey did not use enemas, which should be taken from 5 to 1 times daily during any fast. Pub. by the author, Meadville, Pa.,

and by L. N. Fowler Company, London, Eng.; 5 in. by 7¼ in.; 207 pp.

Pashutin, Victor.

The Director of the Imperial Military Medical Academy, Professor and Academist, Petrograd, Russia.

"Pathological Physiology," a course of General Experimental Pathology (in Russian), 1902, Vol. II, pt. 1, about 1,700 pp. A lengthy discussion of fasting and its effects upon animals and man, of which the first part, about 1,000 pp., has been translated into English by Michel Groosenberg, Russian translator for the Carnegie Institute of Washington, Nutrition Laboratories, and typewritten copies placed in different libraries, including the John Crerar Library of Chicago, and New York Public Library.

Macfadden, B. A. S

Oswald, F., M. D.

"*Fasting, Hydropathy and Exercise,*" 1903.

Shaw, J. Austin.

"*The Best Thing in the World,*" 1906. A diary of a 45-day fast by the author. 125 pp.; 4¼x6½.

Carnegie Institute of Washington, Bull. No. 77, 1907, 542 pp. "The Influence of Inanition on Metabolism," by F. G. Benedict. A lengthy study of short fasts and their effect on metabolism. As few of these fasts were over 7 days in length, and as the body always throws off considerable "refuse" material the first week or two of a fast, the present writer does not consider any of these experiments of sufficient length to measure the true metabolism of the body, and consequently of no value.

Eales, Dr. I. J., M. D., D. O.

"*Healthology,*" 1907.

A description of the author's 31 days' fast with a discussion of the subject written more from the point of view of a fat man who realizes his health is deteriorating and finds in fasting a remedy. Pub. by Dr. I. J. Eales, Chicago, Ill.

Carrington, H. C.

"*Vitality, Fasting and Nutrition,*" 1908. A large volume, one of the most complete and best discussions of the fasting treatment with all its ramifications that the present author has seen; in fact, there is too much for a sick person to grasp or remember until he can use it. More adapted to the use of those who want to make a thorough study of fasting than to those who are sick and willing to try fasting. This is the book which first brought fasting to the present writer's attention about 1908 or 1909, when he was ready to "try anything." 1st Ed. Rebman Company, New York; 6 in. by 9 in.; 648 pp.

Hazzard, Dr. Linda B., D. O.

"*Fasting for the Cure of Disease.*" 1908. Probably the best exposition of the fasting cure for a sick person who wants to have complete directions for a fast; with not too much unnecessary detail. The book (1st Ed.) the present author depended on and followed during practically all his fasting. Now in 3rd Ed. Physical Culture Pub. Co., New York; 5 in. by 7½ in.; 179 pp.

Sinclair, Upton and Michael Williams.

"*Good Health and How We Won It,*" 1909. A discussion of light diet, fresh air, bathing, Fletcherism, meat, etc.; 5 in. by 7½ in.; 300 pp. Pub. F. A. Stokes & Co., New York.

Sinclair, Upton.

"*The Fasting Cure,*" 1911. A small book describing the author's experiences, about 35,000 words. Pub. Michell Kennerly, New York and London; 5 in. by 7½ in.

Wilcox, Van R.

"*Correct Living,*" 1904. An account of the author's 60-day fast and cures obtained.

Guelpa, Dr. G. (Paris).

(Translated by F. S. Arnold) "Autointoxication and Disintoxication"—an account of a new fasting treatment of diabetes and other chronic diseases by very short fasts, generally 3 to 4 days each, about 1912: Rebman & Co., New York; 4½ in. by 7 in.; 152 pp.

Macfadden, B. A., and others.

"*Macfadden's Encyclopedia of Physical Culture.*" 1912, Vol. 3. A very good article of about 96 pages on Fasting.

Carnegie Institute of Washington, Bull. No. 203, 1915.

"A Study of Prolonged Fasting," by F. G. Benedict, 416 pp.

A *strikingly incomplete* resume of some (mostly foreign) prior literature on fasting, and a carefully detailed report of a partial fast of 31 days made by A. Levanzin in hopes of proving the beneficial effects of long, or "complete" fasts to natural hunger.

All the really important prior authorities on fasting, particularly Dr. E. H. Dewey, the discoverer of the fasting treatment for disease, Dr. L. B. Hazzard, who developed the use and importance of the enemas during the fast; each of whom have had experience with several thousand cases of fasting, and Mr. Hereward Carrington, who has written the most complete discussion of the subject in print, are totally ignored, their names not even being mentioned.

This, together with the apparently contemptuous attitude assumed toward them, and the way in which the fast was conducted, violating all the tenets of their teachings, seems to be a grievous slighting of American learning.

All the important results obtainable by fasting were lost; 1st, through not using enemas ("omitted for convenience"), and 2nd, through premature ending of the fast over the energetic protests of Mr. Levanzin, who had a thorough grasp of the importance of fasting until natural hunger returned.

INDEX

CPSIA information can be obtained
at www.ICGtesting.com
Printed in the USA
BVHW092346020922
646137BV00002B/54